Paramedic
Skills
Manual

Paramedic Skills Manual

Second Edition

CHARLES PHILLIPS, M.D.

PHILIP FROMAN, M.D.

CAROL HAGBERG, R.N.

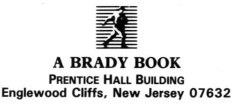

A BRADY BOOK
PRENTICE HALL BUILDING
Englewood Cliffs, New Jersey 07632

Library of Congress Cataloging-in-Publication Data

Phillips, Charles
  Paramedic skills manual / Charles Phillips, Philip Froman, Carol
Hagberg. — 2nd ed.
    p. cm.
  ''A Brady book.''
  ISBN 0-89303-750-8
  1. Emergency medicine—Handbooks, manuals, etc.   2. Emergency
medical technicians. I. Froman, Philip. II. Hagberg, Carol.
III. Title.
RC86.7.P46   1990
616.02′5—dc20   89-22774
                                                           CIP

Art and Photo Credits:

Chapter Opening photographs by Brian Haimar. Figure 2–100 supplied by Ohmeda Emergency
  Care of Orchard Park, New York. Figures 2–64 to 2–81 supplied by International Medical
  Devices, Inc. Figures 7–2, 7–3a and 7–3b supplied by Betty O'Rourke, EMS Director,
  Orange County, CA.

NOTICE

It is the intent of the author and publisher that this skills manual be used as part of a formal EMT paramedic
course taught by a qualified instructor. The care procedures here represent accepted practices in the listed
states. They are not offered as a standard of care. Prehospital level emergency care is to be performed
under the authority and guidance of a licensed physician. It is the reader's responsibility to know and follow
local care protocols as provided by the medical advisors directing the system to which he or she belongs.
Also, it is the reader's responsibility to stay informed of emergency care procedure changes.

Editorial/production supervision and
  interior design: **Lillian Glennon**
Cover design: **Ben Santora**
Manufacturing buyer: **Dave Dickey**

 © 1990, 1980 by Prentice-Hall, Inc.
A Division of Simon & Schuster
Englewood Cliffs, New Jersey 07632

Printed in the United States of America

10 9 8 7 6 5 4 3 2 1

ISBN   0-89303-750-8

PRENTICE-HALL INTERNATIONAL (UK) LIMITED, *London*
PRENTICE-HALL OF AUSTRALIA PTY. LIMITED, *Sydney*
PRENTICE-HALL CANADA INC., *Toronto*
PRENTICE-HALL HISPANOAMERICANA, S.A., *Mexico*
PRENTICE-HALL OF INDIA PRIVATE LIMITED, *New Delhi*
PRENTICE-HALL OF JAPAN, INC., *Tokyo*
SIMON & SCHUSTER, ASIA PTE. LTD., *Singapore*
EDITORA PRENTICE-HALL DO BRASIL, LTDA., *Rio de Janeiro*

Contents

Preface

Writing a book, particularly in my style as an individual working on his own time, is an enormous, two- to three-year project. I find the idea that students will someday use such a text to better understand prehospital care is insufficient to provide the motivation needed. Instead, much of my energy comes from the continuous encouragement of my current students, who have been exposed to the rescue concepts, individual chapters, or early drafts of the book. First of all, then, I thank these students—citizens, EMTs, nurses, paramedics, and physicians—for their enthusiasm, positive suggestions, and thoughtful critiques which kept me going even when the process seemed endless.

I credit much of what I know in the area of priority assessment to Dr. George Degnan, trauma surgeon at Contra Costa County Hospital in Martinez, California. His training in England in both trauma surgery and orthopedics during World War II, under the guidance of some great masters, was crystallized into priceless clinical observations immune from the modern trend toward diagnosis by machine. His ''first principles'' (''pearls'' to medical students) are used throughout this book.

Chief Jerry Fender, training officer for the large Consolidated Fire Department in Concord, California, has been my principal tutor in skills organization, description, and competency testing. His careful reading and review led to the development of the many procedure guides in the manual.

Once the book took formal shape in an early draft, I sought reviews from experts like Cathy Mickelberry, R.N., Shelly Fredrickson, R.N., Sandy Kennedy, R.N., and Donna Brandstrom, R.N. Ms. Brandstrom in particular wrote an exhaustive critique based on 10 years' experience as an emergency department supervisor, five years' experience as supervisor of a combined intensive care unit and coronary care unit, and one year's experience as a full-time paramedic coordinator.

Next I approached the San Francisco Bay Area Paramedic Task Force and MICN (Mobile Intensive Care Nurse) Task Force for regional input. Reviews were obtained from such experts as Paramedic Andy Yaffe of San Francisco; Santa Clara County Paramedic Coordinator

Peggy Burroughs, R.N.; Marin County Paramedic Coordinator Barbara Foster, R.N.; and Stanford Prehospital Care Coordinator Barbara Secord, R.N. Ms. Burroughs and Ms. Secord wrote excellent, extensive reviews. Ms. Burroughs has ridden out with paramedics on over 1000 Code 3 runs. Ms. Secord added the expertise gained in her experience as an MICN in San Diego's program in southern California.

Al Belski, Acquisitions Editor with the Brady Company at the initiation of the publishing process, started the first national review of the book now officially titled *Paramedic Skills Manual.* Contributors included Gail Walraven, R.N., Lou Jordan, P.A., and Karen Campbell, R.N. These national experts pointed out areas to be further developed. Ms. Walraven, in particular, helped clarify the audience of the book and the need to separate out excess theory material.

Rick Weimer, Mr. Belski's successor, took the book, now revised once again, to yet another group of national reviewers, including Linda Gericke, R.N., Edward Hoffer, M.D., Midge Moreau, R.N., and Valentino Menis, M.D. The book was then passed into the full production phase.

Marlise Reidenbach was the production editor assigned to the book. Her interest and enthusiasm ensured that no corners were cut that might sacrifice clarity of presentation. Decisions were made with the goal of having a text which catered to the needs of the paramedic student ready to assimilate new information and embark on a new career.

Rick Brady flew out to California for a concentrated eight solid days of photography, resulting in 600 photographs of paramedic skill sequences. His previous experience made him a co-creator in many areas. His interest kept the author from yielding to the temptation to take shortcuts simply out of fatigue. The result is a highly pictorial book with a unique and large color slide collection as a companion service to the instructor. Many others participated in an initial series used for reference photos.

The following paramedics participated as models for the photography: Dave Brown, Larry Chaney, Brenda Garcia, Rob Goodyear, Robert Lunardini, and Rick Todd. EMTs from the Moraga Fire Department also helped, as did models Ronnie Atkinson, Melissa Bruner, Guy Fitch, Elise Johnson, Henry Mailer, Jennifer Robertson, and Patricia Wolfman.

Don Sellers, art director and medical illustrator (AMI) for the Brady Company, headed a team of artists to illustrate numerous key points in the book. His background as a paramedic, as well as his experience as the art director/illustrator of over 100 books, resulted in the quality evidenced in the book. His willingness to perfect drawings even to the smallest detail is witnessed throughout the book.

Many others contributed heavily to a book that is surely a team effort even though initiated by a single author. I hope they will find the book worthy of their efforts.

Our thanks to the following people whose comments helped shape the book:

1. M. Charlotte Yeager, R.N., of Doylestown, Pennsylvania

2. Robert H. Gaumer of Harrisburg, Pennsylvania

3. Debby Pavy, REMT-P, of Oklahoma City, Oklahoma

4. Al D. Hudson of Chapel Hill, North Carolina

5. Michael Olds of Baltimore, Maryland

6. Carolyn Schmidt of Little Rock, Arkansas

7. David Ranson of Cheyenne, Wyoming

The following reviewers, utilized by the Brady Company, were diligent in seeing to it that the skills book was updated in content but not disturbed in focus:

1. Paul A. Berlin of Gig Harbor, Washington

2. James L. Paturas of Bridgeport, Connecticut

3. Bruce R. Shode of Cleveland, Ohio

4. Bryan E. Bledsoe, D.O., of Odessa, Texas

Charles Phillips, M. D.
Philip Froman, M. D.
Carol Hagberg, R. N.

About the Authors

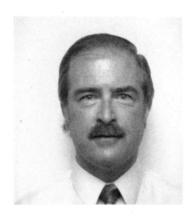

Dr. Charles Phillips

Dr. Phillips has spent the last twenty years providing direct, critical care to patients in a variety of settings—emergency departments, intensive care units, and coronary care units. He has also assisted in numerous life saving operations in the surgical suites of trauma centers. He is Board Certified in Emergency Medicine and has been a member of the American College of Emergency Physicians.

Dr. Phillips is currently the Director of Emergency Medicine at the King Faisal Specialist Hospital and Research Centre in Riyadh, Saudi Arabia. His duties include providing supervision of on site emergency care for the King of Saudi Arabia. Paramedics are part of the hospital EMS teams.

His multiple books in emergency care have been a spinoff of his intense interest in teaching. He has taught full EMS courses to citizens, EMTs, paramedics, nurses, and physicians. He has additionally provided problem solving consultations to several EMS regions involving several million people. He has taught EMS in the United States, New Zealand, and Saudi Arabia.

His overall teaching goal is to provide a priority system that is appropriate at all levels of EMS so that communication is easy and clear. His A-G priority system provides such a common language and is the organizing principle of this book.

Dr. Phillips is currently Head of Emergency Services for the King Faisol Specialist Hospital in Saudi Arabia. He also works with paramedics, and is the Director of the Life Support Training Center.

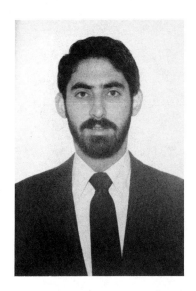

Philip J. Froman, M.D.
Paramedic Instructor

Philip Froman graduated from Daniel Freeman Paramedic School in 1979, first in class standing. He attended the University of California, Santa Barbara and graduated with a Bachelor of Arts in Law and Society. During his years at UCSB he worked first as an EMT and then as a paramedic with the UC Santa Barbara Police Department, Paramedic Rescue Division. After graduation, Philip worked with a private ambulance service in the Sierras before taking a position as Director of Rescue Services with the Penn Valley Fire Department. During this period he was also on the faculty at two colleges, teaching in the EMT program.

Philip is currently a first year Emergency Medicine Resident at Wright State University affiliated program in Dayton, Ohio after graduating from the University of California Los Angeles, School of Medicine. While attending medical school he also taught EMT classes at UCLA and Paramedic courses at Daniel Freeman Medical Center. He was also involved in prehospital care and emergency medicine research at UCLA and Olive View Medical Centers.

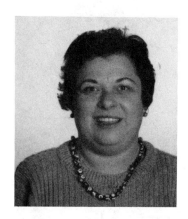

Carol Hagberg—R.N., MICN, J.D.

Carol Hagberg has worked in critical care areas: intensive care units, coronary care units, and emergency departments continuously over the past two decades. In 1969 she was a staff nurse at Harbor General Hospital's CCU when J. Michael Criley, M.D. began first training Los Angeles County firefighters as paramedics. Since that time she has been involved with Los Angeles County Prehospital care in a variety of capacities.

As a paramedic instructor for the county, she taught paramedics, and initiated the first MICN development course and base hospital physician training program. In 1975 she helped organize the Paramedic Services Section of the Los Angeles EMSA and served as assistant Chief of Prehospital Care and Chief of the Emergency Aid Plan.

Joining Daniel Freeman Hospital Paramedic Training Program as course coordinator in the spring of 1979, she continues to train paramedics and EMT-Basics on a continuous basis. Receiving her J.D. from Western State University College of Law, her ultimate goal is to combine her nursing and legal backgrounds and practice EMS law.

She attended the Long Beach City College R.N. program and has a B.A. from Long Beach State College. She is currently certified as an MICN for Los Angeles County and is a member of ENA.

Introduction

PURPOSE

There are many thousand *emergency medical technician paramedics* (EMT-Ps) performing prehospital advanced life-support skills in the United States and throughout the world at this time. These paramedics are bringing emergency department skills to the patient at home and in the street. As more paramedic programs are starting every year, it is clear that this new rescue professional is here to stay. It is now appropriate to standardize the training and testing of the paramedic. This will provide national mobility for the paramedic and help the hundreds of paramedic programs achieve common objectives. This skills manual is designed to standardize the skill training and skill testing of paramedics nationally and internationally. Some of the skills are used by EMT-Intermediates. In some EMS systems, EMT-Basic students are taught selected advanced skills as well and can use this book.

STUDENT MANUAL

The manual has been prepared with detailed drawings and photographs, so that it may be used by the student throughout a paramedic course as a training guide. A test for each skill is also defined. It is the intent of the author that each student be given the manual at the beginning of a paramedic course. At the point of final skill testing, the principal "surprise" will be *which* of these skills will be tested and under what conditions of stress. The manual should have equal value for paramedic continuing education and refresher courses, particularly where skill utilization in the field is infrequent and review is needed. Also, hospitals, that are separate from training institutions and are responsible for paramedic skill maintenance, may use the manual as a guide to skill level.

NOT A TEXTBOOK

The skills manual is not a textbook that tries to get at the "when and why" to do a skill. It is much more of a "how to do it" book. Each chapter presents only a small amount of background material which directly relates to or enhances the skill presented. A standard didactic text should be used to define the "when and why" issues.

INSTRUCTIONAL STRATEGY

Often, courses are budgeted for the lecture style and rarely have sufficient time allowed or equipment purchased for good lab sessions. In the area of emergency medicine this can be particularly disastrous, especially at the more advanced levels, where equipment is more complicated. The authors believe that courses for rescue personnel should be constructed so that there is at least one piece of equipment for every four students during any "lab." In a paramedic course this should be true as well. The instructor cannot depend on the "clinical" or inhospital portion of the course to teach skills, since each hospital and each clinical instructor may teach skill differently, and standardization becomes impossible. Continuing education then becomes even more difficult, since there is no way to review a skill not originally defined. Good skill performance should be attained, at least on manikins, before students start the clinical phase.

SKILL SELECTION

The skills selected have in general been nationally and internationally accepted as paramedic skills. Where there might be a debate concerning the effectiveness of two skills, as for example the endotracheal intubation versus esophageal obturator airway, both skills are presented. The area of skill selection has been pioneered by both the National Academy of Sciences and Nancy Caroline, M.D., formerly of the University of Pittsburgh. The Advanced Cardiac Life Support programs of the American Heart Association and the Advanced Trauma Life Support courses of the American College of Surgeons have also helped to create uniformity of skills. Even though some skills are restricted by certain EMS systems, they are presented for completeness. Instructors will make selections as needed and point out the limitations of local laws. Skills added in this second edition include use of oxygen/nitrous oxide combinations, the Nu-Trach and Pedia-Trach for cricothyrotomy, and external pacing of the heart.

SKILL LEVEL

Most programs have accepted the requirement that a student coming into a paramedic course should have mastered basic life-support emergency medical technician skills. The senior author has written a text *(Basic Life Support: Skills Manual*, second edition) at the basic level, including the noninvasive skills of oral airway insertion, positive pressure breathing, control of bleeding, CPR, wound care, spine and extremity splinting, emergency childbirth, control of violence, and basic communications. *These skills will not be repeated in the manual.* Instead, the advanced skills covered in this manual are those which are generally invasive — long airway tubes, intravenous solutions and drugs, defibrillation, and so forth. Shock trousers, although not invasive, are covered in this manual.

PRIORITY ORGANIZATION

The key to dealing with patients with either multiple-system trauma or severe medical decompensation is the use of an expanded ABC priority system. These priorities are listed in the order in which they must be evaluated and resolved.

*Airway** — Is there an open passageway for respiration?
Breathing — Are the mechanics of air exchange adequate?
Circulation — Are vital organs being perfused?
Delicate CNS — Is there a threat to the brain or cord?
External soft tissue — Is there an external soft tissue injury?
Fracture — Is there skeletal instability?
GI/GU† — Is there nonbleeding abdominal/pelvic distress?

Using this system, the rescuer will know that a tension pneumothorax (B priority) will take priority over an open leg fracture (E and F priority). As with the basic skills manual, this advanced skills manual uses the A-to-G sequence for chapter order. Instructors are encouraged to use the book in sequence to reinforce the system rather than isolating such topics as "medical emergencies."

SKILL FORMAT

A skill properly presented includes an introduction, indications, precautions, equipment, discussion of how to do it, and then an explanation of how to test it. The skill test is defined in terms of the skill, performance, conditions, and standard. An example is as follows:

Skill	Shock Trousers
Performance	Demonstrate how to put on, inflate, maintain, and deflate a pair of shock trousers.
Conditions	1. Simulated patient is in shock due to ruptured ectopic pregnancy.
	2. Vital signs: BP 80/40 and pulse 120; foot pulses are present and motor function plus sensation is intact.
	3. Shock trousers are available in manufacturer's container next to patient.
	4. Base hospital has authorized rescuer to put shock trousers on patient.
	5. Rescuer is positioned 5 feet from patient until told "you may begin."
Standard	1. Rescuer identifies himself and reassures patient.
	2. Orally assess the condition: "The patient has probable hypovolemic shock."
	3. Place shock trousers between the patient's legs.
	4. Lift patient's legs as trousers are brought up to a snug groin fit.
	5. Etc.

In this way the student is aware of the skill and the method of testing proficiency. During an actual test, the information under the headings "Skill," "Performance," and

---

*Any airway skills to be performed on the trauma patient must be performed always keeping in mind the possibility of a broken neck.
†GI/GU stands for gastrointestinal/genitourinary.

"Conditions" can be copied and handed to students to read before starting. The verbal assessment step has been added to the second edition, reflecting an evolution in EMS communications in the 1980s.

STANDARDIZED SKILL LISTING

The following skills are covered in this manual and represent about 90% of a possible paramedic course. The remaining 10% should be the perogative of the instructor and reflect local needs: for example, snake bite, decompression sickness, and so forth.

1. *Patient Evaluation*
   Advanced patient evaluation

2. *Airway Skills*
   Esophageal obturator airway insertion
   Adult endotracheal intubation
   Infant endotracheal intubation
   Endotracheal suctioning
   Percutaneous cricothyrotomy
   Surgical cricothyrotomy
   Inhalation analgesia (nitrous oxide)

3. *Breathing Skills*
   Pleural decompression
   Percutaneous transtracheal ventilation

4. *Circulation Skills*
   Antishock trousers
   Trauma IV

5. *Medication Administration*
   Subcutaneous injection
   Intramuscular injection
   Intravenous preload bolus
      administration
   Intravenous piggyback drip
   Endotracheal medication administration
   Drip rate calculation
   Inhalation analgesia

6. *Dysrhythmias*
   Application of monitor electrodes
   Paper readout
   Rhythm interpretation
   Carotid sinus massage
   Two-minute CPR
   Defibrillation
   Cardioversion
   Pacemaker magnet
   Noninvasive external pacing

7. *Advanced Communications*

CONCLUSION

The total skill sequence then follows the A-to-G priority order, although basic skills such as splinting are not repeated. Skills dealing with the unresponsive patient are a mix of skills from various chapters and therefore are not separately described.

Utilization of advanced skills should not proceed simply from self-study of this manual. Instead, the student should develop the techniques under supervision in class, then in the hospital, and finally in the field. Final permission to use the skill comes from a physician directly or indirectly, exercising medical control within a coordinated emergency medical system.

Paramedic
Skills
Manual

1

Patient Evaluation

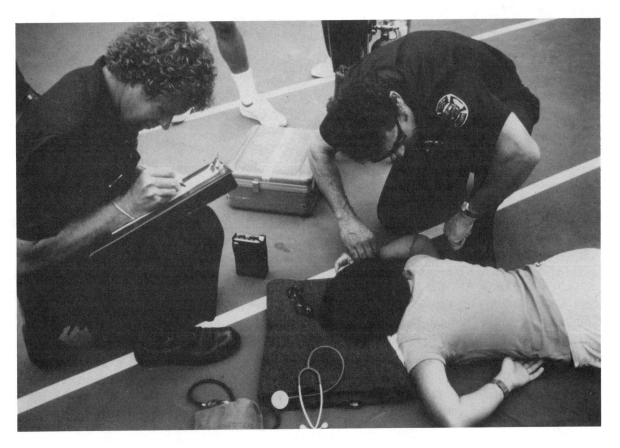

Skills Objectives

- **Advanced Patient Evaluation**—Demonstrate how to complete an advanced-level patient evaluation, including the four parts of the SOAP process:

  a. *Subjective* interview to search for symptoms

  b. *Objective* examination to search for signs

  c. *Assessment* of probable emergency condition present

  d. *Plan* of treatment to restore health

Outline

Patient Evaluation Skills Description

INTRODUCTION

Patient evaluation is the cornerstone of appropriate prehospital medical care. A paramedic should choose skills *after*, not *before*, patient evaluation, if utilized. Even in the dramatic situation of cardiopulmonary arrest, inquiry about traumatic versus non-traumatic (medical) origin and examination of airway, breathing, and circulation precedes the major treatment step of CPR (cardiopulmonary resuscitation; discussed in Chapter 6), whether basic or advanced.

Little is gained by applying the wrong intervention, however skillfully, if the patient evaluation is incorrect. Because patient evaluation is the first logical step in patient care, it is a natural first chapter for a skills manual.

Most of the early rescue textbooks developed different patient evaluation for every condition; for example, ''. . . in case of a burn look for . . . .'' But a good evaluation should be used to *discover a condition rather than confirm it*. The paramedic needs one thorough, advanced examination that proceeds in a logical pattern, resistant to distraction, uncovering all important findings needed to make good prehospital treatment decisions.

Paramedic versus EMT-Basic Patient Evaluation

Most students using this book have first completed a more basic emergency medical technician course. During such training, patient evaluation skills were learned. The EMT-paramedic level evaluation, in contrast to that of the EMT-Basic, expands mostly the area of patient interview. The physical examination of the patient is quite similar. An example of expanded interview occurs in the evaluation of shortness of breath. The EMT is encouraged to ask one or two questions, whereas the paramedic is more likely to ask about seven. Such detail relates to treatment options—the EMT deciding positioning and whether or not to use oxygen, while the paramedic may consider a variety of medications.

The SOAP Evaluation System

Regardless of the condition, the four steps of patient evaluation are: subjective interview, objective exam, assessment of the problem, and plan of treatment (Figure 1.1). The letters SOAP summarize these steps.* The SOAP evaluation process is being used in almost every medical school in the country and has been incorporated into many active prehospital care systems as well. Throughout this chapter, each of the sub-

*SOAP is a memory device. The uses of SOAP and others, such as PQRST, PAST MED, and AEIOU tips, are given as a means to help students retain the information for learning purposes, not to replace the learning itself.

headings of this schematic is discussed. Then the flexibility of the SOAP approach is presented. This process will avoid the usual division of a *trauma exam* or a *medical exam*, each of which can lead to tunnel vision. Such exams should really be expansions of a comprehensive approach appropriate to all patients.

The new National Curriculum for paramedics has been formally published. It appears that the paramedic will be taught patient evaluation as a fourfold process: primary evaluation, resuscitation, secondary evaluation, and packaging. The integration of this with the three patient surveys and the SOAP system is shown in Figure 1.2.

Thus primary evaluation combines a primary survey and vital signs. This is appropriate, since in most cases the paramedic team is evaluating both classic ABC signs of life—the primary survey—and the vital signs simultaneously. A particular resuscitation step such as applying antishock garments (ASG or MAST) might be chosen either from the primary survey finding of traumatic arrest or the vital signs finding of a blood pressure of 50/30.

SOAP
Subjective Interview
Objective Examination
Assessment of Problems
Plan of Treatment

Figure 1-1 SOAP system.

	PRIMARY SURVEY		VITAL SIGNS	SECONDARY SURVEY
Subjective interview	1. Primary evaluation		3. Secondary evaluation	
Objective examination				
Assessment of problem	2. Resuscitation of patient		4. Packaging patient	
Plan of treatment				

Figure 1-2 Patient evaluation in four phases per the new National Paramedic Curriculum.

Patient Evaluation

Patient evaluation will be separated into the four elements of the SOAP examination: subjective interview, objective exam, assessment of problem, and plan of action. Each is discussed in turn.

SUBJECTIVE INTERVIEW

The subjective interview is the first part of patient evaluation. The interview includes reports from the first responders; information provided by observers, friends, or relatives; and symptoms of the patient. The goal is to organize the material gathered into the following categories:

> *Chief complaint*—principal problem triggering the call for help (e.g., ''chest pain for thirty minutes'')
>
> *History of present illness (HPI)*—background of the chief complaint (e.g., previous heart attacks)
>
> *Past medical history (PMH)*—pertinent illnesses, medications, and medication allergies

As seen in Figure 1.3, these are organized in the order just presented. If time is very limited—as with the life-and-death situation—at least a chief complaint will be obtained.

Some of the specific questions to ask the first responder and the patient are presented in Table 1.1. The purpose of asking the questions is discussed as well.

Alert Patient

The alert patient can be interviewed in the standard format shown in Table 1.1. The interview system can be used in this sequence for almost any alert patient. If the patient is a small child, the mother is interviewed. The interview of patients with two common symptons—shortness of breath (dyspnea) and chest pain—are expanded below.

PAST MEDICAL HISTORY (FOR DYSPNEA). Dyspnea is approached as an acute episode and underlying chronic condition using the following PAST MED memory aid:

* *Acute*
  Progression of symptoms
  Associated chest pain
  Sputum change
  Tiredness

* *Chronic*
  Medications
  Exercise tolerance
  Diagnosis last time

PQRST FOR CHEST PAIN. The PQRST system seen in Table 1.1 is especially suited

PATIENT EVALUATION			
	Life/Death	Critical	Serious
S	Chief Complaint	History of present illness	Past medical history
O			
A			
P			

Figure 1–3

Table 1.1. INTERVIEW FORMAT (ALERT PATIENT).

Type of Question	Example of Question	Example of Answer
1. Introduction (includes reassurance and permission to treat)	I am paramedic Bill Smith. I am here to help you. What is your name?	My name is Jim Clark.
2. Chief complaint	What problem are you having?	I got this sudden chest pain while driving.
3. History of present illness (PQRST system)[a]	*Provocation?* *Palliative?* What were you doing just before the pain started?	I was driving along and started worrying about bills.
	Quality/Quantity? What does it feel like? Any sweating, nausea, or shortness of breath? What relieves the pain?	It's like a tight band around my chest. I sweated profusely.
	Radiation?/Region? Where else does it go?	It went down my left arm and up into my jaw.
	Severity? How bad is it on a scale of 1 to 10?	It's one of the worst pains I've ever had. A 10.
	Timing? How long has it lasted? Have you had it before?	It's been almost an hour. It's easing off some now. I had it once before.
4. Age	How old are you?	I am 55.
5. Past health	Are you under a doctor's care for anything?	Yes, angina.
6. Current medications	Do you take any prescription drugs?	Nitroglycerin, but I left it at home.
7. Allergies	Are you allergic to any drugs?	I get hives with Lasix.

[a]The PQRST system of interviewing has been credited to Ron Stewart, M.D.

to chest pain. It can also be used for patients with abdominal pain. The paramedic should be encouraged to recognize abdominal *bleeding* as the chief *prehospital* priority issue in the abdominal–pelvic cavity: for example, bleeding ulcer, ruptured abdominal aortic aneurysm, bleeding ectopic pregnancy, bleeding spleen, and bleeding from pelvic fracture.

Unconscious Patient

Similar information must be elicited for the unconscious patient when necessary. The paramedic will often interview relatives, friends, or witnesses in these cases to get a good picture of the patient's subjective complaints. Unconscious patient possibilities are best recalled through the memory aid developed around AEIOU and TIPS:

> A—Alcohol, apnea, arrhythmia
>
> E—Epilepsy
>
> I—Insulin (hypo- or hyperglycemia)
>
> O—Overdose
>
> U—Underdose (too little cortisone, thyroxin, etc.), uremia (metabolic conditions)
>
> T—Trauma, tumor
>
> I—Infection
>
> P—Psychiatric
>
> S—Stroke (cardiovascular emergencies)

Trauma Patient

In the case of trauma, the subjective interview is just as important. Although the subjective complaint may appear obvious, a complete subjective interview should be conducted. A thorough evaluation of mechanism of injury (auto versus auto) and the results of the injury (a bent steering wheel and cracked windshield) should be included.

OBJECTIVE EXAMINATION

The objective examination consists of a search for signs of health or illness. A *symptom* is something felt by the patient, whereas a *sign* is a finding observed by the EMT, such as pallor or a fast pulse.

A common approach to the objective examination is to divide it into primary and secondary surveys. The primary survey deals with life and death issues, whereas the secondary survey is a search for injury. There is much disagreement as to where the vital signs fit into this scheme.

An effective system is the division of the objective examination into three principal steps:

> *Primary survey*—exam for *presence* of life-and-death priorities
>
> *Vital signs*—exam for the *quality* of life-and-death priorities
>
> *Secondary survey*—head-to-toe search for injury

The primary survey, then, is really a priority survey.

The A-to-G system is a memonic device that categorizes all of the body tissues so that their relative importance or priority is understood (see Figure 1.4). When faced with the multiply injured patient, the paramedic needs to organize and treat these injuries in priority order. The A-to-G system in summary is as follows:

> *Airway*—passageway for respiration
>
> *Breathing*—mechanics of respiration
>
> *Circulation*—perfusion of vital organs
>
> *Delicate CNS*—brain and cord
>
> *External soft tissue*—skin, peripheral circulation + nerves
>
> *Fracture*—long bone or joint injury
>
> *GI/GU*—nonbleeding abdominal–pelvic condition

Primary and intermediate survey focuses on the A-to-D priorities as they determine life and death.

Thus the objective examination will be discussed in three sections corresponding to the three surveys summarized in Figure 1.5. Note that in the field situation the objective examination may be completed by two rescuers working together; one does the primary and secondary survey while the other obtains vital signs.

EVOLUTION OF
PRIORITIES IN MEDICAL RESCUE

1950s—Red Cross (AB's)
  Airway
  Bleeding
  Shock

1960s—American Heart Association (ABC)
  Airway
  Breathing
  Circulation

1970s—Rescue Instructors (ABC's)
  Airway
  Breathing
  Circulation
  Shock

1975—Ron Stewart, M.D. (ABC's)
  Airway
  Breathing
  Circulation
  Sugar and spine

*1980s—American College of
  Surgeons (A–E)*
  Airway/C-spine
  Breathing
  Circulation
  Disability (CNS)
  Expose (to examine)

1985—Full Body System (A–G)
  Airway (protecting C-spine)
  Breathing
  Circulation
  Delicate CNS*
  External soft tissue
  Fracture
  GI/GU† nonbleeding

*CNS, Central nervous system—brain and spinal cord (in contrast to the peripheral nervous system, consisting of nerves)
†GI/GU, gastrointestinal and genitourinary systems.

Figure 1–4   The evolution of priorities in medical rescue.

PATIENT EVALUATION

	Life/Death	Critical	Serious
S			
O	Primary survey A ↘ D	Vital signs A ↘ D	Secondary survey Head ↘ Toe
A			
P			

Figure 1–5   A summary of the objective examination.

Primary Survey

The goal of the primary survey, then, is to search for the presence of life. Is the airway open? Is there breathing as determined by air and/or chest movement? Is there a pulse or site of rapid bleeding—circulation issues? Is the patient responsive to voice or pain—delicate CNS issues? In case of any head or neck trauma, suspect cervical spine injury until proven otherwise by x-ray.

Although the general approach in patient evaluation is to finish the exam before treating, certain findings during the primary survey lead to emergency assessments requiring immediate treatment. These are presented along with the examination steps.

Step 1—Examine the Airway

Exam Step	Common Findings	Emergency Assessments	Skill Applied[a]
• Pinch trapezius muscles gently without moving neck.	Combined gurgling/snoring sounds	Partial airway obstruction	Chin lift maneuvers (Figure 1.6)
	(*or*)	(*or*)	(*or*)
• Listen at the mouth for sounds of obstruction.	No sound and no movement of exhaled air	Complete airway obstruction	Trial mouth-to-mouth ventilation (Figure 1.7)
• Feel for exhaled air.			

[a]In case of trauma assume cervical fracture—thus chin lift is chosen over head tilt.

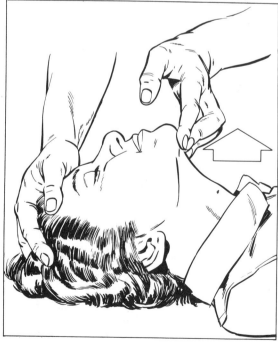

Figure 1–6   The head-tilt, chin-lift maneuver.

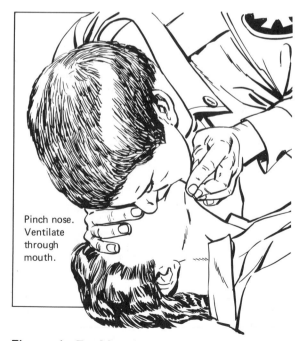

Pinch nose. Ventilate through mouth.

Figure 1–7   Mouth to mouth ventilation.

Step 2—Check for Breathing

Exam Step	Common Findings	Emergency Assessments	Skills Applied
• Listen for the sounds of air exhalation after airway cleared. • Check skin color.	Poor ventilation exchange and cyanosis (blue discoloration of the skin) (*or*) Apnea (no breathing) (*or*)	Hypoventilation (inadequate air exchange) and hypoxia (low body oxygen) (*or*) Apnea (*or*)	Assist ventilation and supplement oxygen (Figures 1.8 and 1.9) (*or*) Ventilate (*or*)
• Check for open chest wound.	Sucking chest wound	Sucking chest wound with risk of tension pneumothorax	Cover open chest wound

For more details, see Chapter 3.

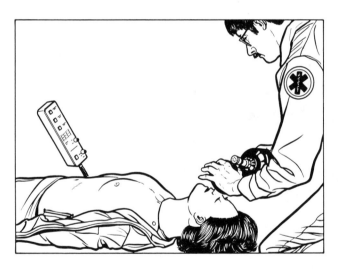

Figure 1–8   Bag valve mask. Assist ventilation.

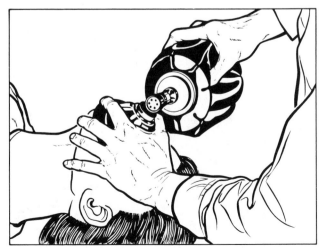

Figure 1–9   Ventilate patient.

Step 3—Examine the Circulation

Exam Step	Common Findings	Emergency Assessments	Skills Applied
• Check major pulses. • Check for active bleeding.	Weak pulses in combination with bleeding (*or*) Absent pulse	Shock from blood loss (*or*) Cardiac arrest	Stop bleeding Treat for shock (*or*) (Figures 1.10 and 1.11) (*or*) Start CPR (See Chapter 6)

For more details, see Chapter 4.

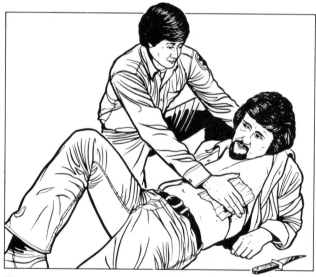

Figure 1–10   Stop bleeding.

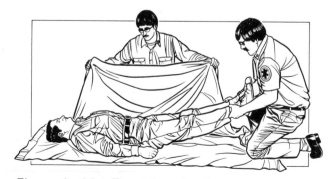

Figure 1–11   Treat for shock.

Step 4—Observe the Delicate CNS

Note: Remember that "delicate CNS" means delicate central nervous system and includes the brain and spinal cord. The less delicate and partially repairable nervous tissue is the peripheral nervous system.

Exam Step	Common Findings	Emergency Assessments	Skills Applied
• Test for responsiveness.	AVPU[a] Alert Verbal response Pain response Unresponsive	Probable traumatic unconsciousness	Keep airway clear; compare status against repeat exams
• Test for posterior midline neck tenderness.	Assume possible cervical fracture if patient is unconscious	Possible cervical fracture	Apply manual traction and cervical collar (Figures 1.12 and 1.13)

[a]This is the AVPU system published by the American College of Surgeons in 1980 in their *Advanced Trauma Life Support Manual.*

For more details, see Chapter 7.

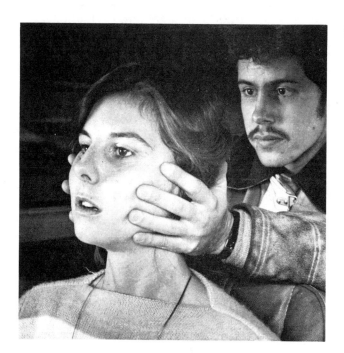

Figure 1–13   Apply stiff collar.

Figure 1–12   Support neck.

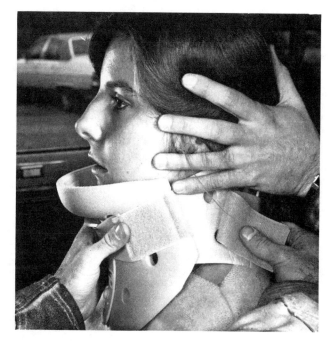

To communicate a primary survey, the student should first practice trying to describe someone who is not ill (Figure 1.14). A description of general health would be as follows:

> The patient has quiet, unlabored respirations. There is no sign of external bleeding. The patient is alert, moving all four extremities.

Obviously, this is too long for the radio. However, it should be learned at this time. In Chapter 7, a shorter version is described. In the case of the second example, the patient described is in moderate distress and the location of the organ system in distress has been identified.

> Patient is alert, is in moderate respiratory distress with labored respirations, but without wounds, bleeding, or deformity.

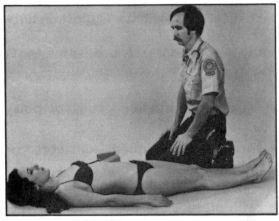

Figure 1–14   Overview.

SUMMARY. Thus the primary survey checks for the *presence* of the A-to-D priorities:

> *Airway*—open, partial obstructed, completely obstructed
>
> *Breathing*—normal, labored, absent
>
> *Circulation*—pulse present, bleeding present

Delicate CNS—responsiveness per AVPU system

To sustain life, immediate treatment intervention is often needed if one of these priorities is absent or at grave risk.

Vital Signs

The vital signs step consists of a brief exam of the *quality* of the various medical priorities. The exam consists of the following steps:

> *Airway*—Listen for noise as evidence of obstruction.
>
> *Breathing*—Check depth, rate, and general effort.
>
> *Circulation*—Check blood pressure and pulse.
>
> *Delicate CNS*—Check level of consciousness to stimuli such as voice, touch, or pain (evaluate with initial patient contact and may be further evaluated if abnormality is present).

Review of Technique

The hospital use of the term "vital signs" refers to blood pressure and TPR (temperature, pulse, and respiration). The temperature in the prehospital setting is usually estimated and mentioned only if high. Therefore, the vital signs for the paramedic in the field are comprised of respiration, blood pressure, and pulse.

Vital signs can change rapidly and should be considered as a baseline to be repeated. Vital signs can often change with positioning; for example, a patient with initial stages of shock may have normal vital signs while lying down, but with sitting his blood pressure will drop and his pulse rate will rise. This would be referred to as postural hypotension. The normal method for taking vital signs will be reviewed and some other variations discussed.

Use Appropriate Terminology

Learning specific terminology such as "There is no tenderness on compression of the chest" also allows the paramedic to communicate clearly to the physician. Such a phrase makes the physician more confident that a good exam was done rather than hearing the alternative: "The chest is negative."

During the testing of this skill, it is necessary to have the rescuer verbalize the terminology; this is one of the reasons the classroom evaluation takes seven minutes. The purpose of this verbalization in class is to be sure that the rescuer is doing the right exam step for the right purpose and to hear that the correct terms are being used. The testing sequence suggests that such terms may be used between two rescuers to communicate the exam as well.

STEP	SPECIFIC MOTION
1. Check respiration and pulse. (Figure 1.15).	Watch respirations for 15 seconds and multiply by 4. Find radial pulse count for 15 seconds and multiply by 4.*
Terminology:	"Respirations are 16 with good tidal volume and not labored. The pulse is 80, strong, and regular."
2. Put on BP cuff (Figure 1.16).	Place BP cuff at least 1 inch above elbow crease. It must be secure.**
Terminology: None.	

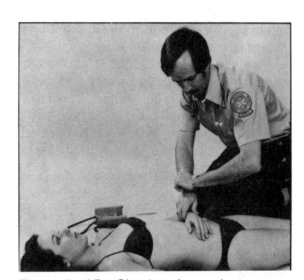

Figure 1–15   Check pulse and respiration.

*If a pulse is irregular, it should be counted for 30 seconds and compared with an apical pulse.

**To determine proper cuff size: The width of the cuff should be approximately two-thirds the length of the arm. If too small, the reading will be falsely high; if too large, the reading will be falsely low.

Blanch test for pediatrics: Elevate extremity and inflate cuff until color change noted on palm of hand. Slowly release cuff pressure and note reading when color returns to palm of hand preinflation color.

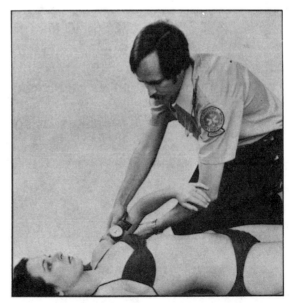

Figure 1–16   Secure blood pressure cuff.

STEP	SPECIFIC MOTION

continued

3. Check palpable BP (systolic estimate in case of noise); Figure 1.17).

Palpate radial pulse† and inflate cuff until pulse disappears; then go 20 points higher; slowly deflate until pulse is felt, then fully deflate cuff.

Terminology: ''The palpable BP is 116.''

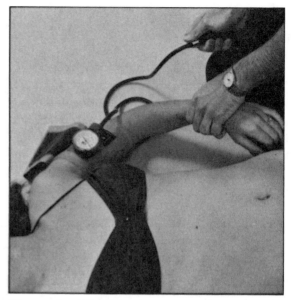

Figure 1–17   Obtain palpable blood pressure.

4. Prepare for full (auscultatory) BP.

Place stethoscope around neck with earpieces facing forward (Figure 1.18).

Terminology: None.

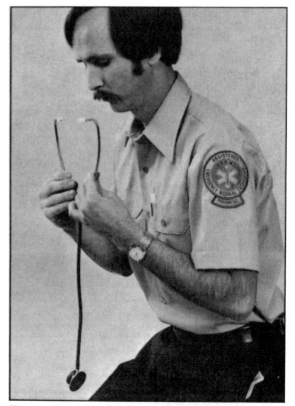

†Some critical care experts prefer to use the brachial pulse with a palpable blood pressure for patients in shock, as the radial pulse disappears at a blood pressure of about 80.

Figure 1–18   Put on stethoscope.

STEP	SPECIFIC MOTION

continued

5. Check full BP.
Palpate brachial artery (Figure 1.19); place diaphragm of stethoscope over brachial artery (Figure 1.20). Inflate cuff to 20 points above palpable BP and slowly deflate. After the systolic and diastolic readings are noted, the cuff is left on the arm in case the BP needs to be rechecked.*

Terminology: ''The blood pressure is 120/80.''

*The blood pressure cuff may be left in place for several reasons: (1) for reassessment later, and (2) as a venous tourniquet for starting an IV (intravenous drip of fluid).

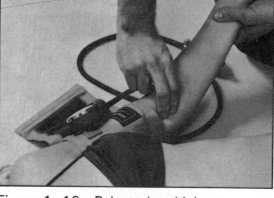

Figure 1–19   Palpate brachial artery.

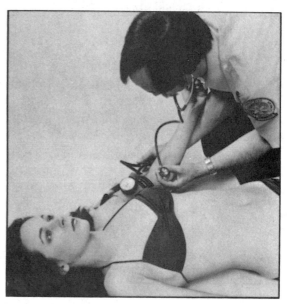

Figure 1–20   Check full blood pressure.

When the paramedic goes on the radio, the patient presentation must be much shorter. This will involve not only selecting those findings that are abnormal, such as a ''deformity of the tibia,'' but also choosing a *pertinent negative* such as ''but with an intact pedal pulse.'' Selection of pertinent negatives will come with experience. Radio communication is discussed in Chapter 7.

Secondary Survey (Head to Toe)

The head-to-toe examination is organized so that there is a specific finding to be sought in each location of the body examined (Figure 1.21). For example, the facial bones are not just randomly examined but are checked for tenderness. This type of goal-

PATIENT EXAMINATION			
	Life/Death	Critical	Serious
S	Chief complaint	History of present illness	PMH Meds Allergies
O	Primary survey A ⟶ D	Vital signs A ⟶ E	Secondary survey Head ⟶ Toe

Figure 1-21

oriented exam resists distractions such as noise, flashing lights, and so on.

Ideally, one might be willing to accept any exam sequence as long as it covered every point. From a practical basis going head to toe, front to back, becomes the most likely exam sequence to be complete and therefore is the format used in this manual. (Remember that in a small, non-critical child, the exam goes foot to head to build the patient's confidence.

It must be remembered that some steps in the survey are optional and that in some cases (a critical patient with a gunshot wound, for example) some parts of the survey may be eliminated to expedite treatment and transport.

STEP	SPECIFIC MOTION
1. Scalp	Palpate hair and scalp for active bleeding (Figure 1.22). At the same time feel any skull deformities. Do not move the neck at all.

Terminology: "The scalp is not bleeding and the skull shows no deformity."

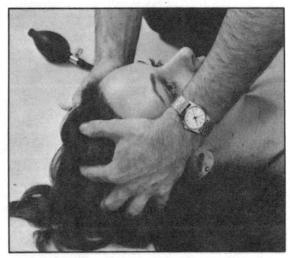

Figure 1-22 Palpate the scalp.

STEP	SPECIFIC MOTION

continued

2. Forehead   Touch the forehead with the back of your hand (Figure 1.23). Note both moisture and temperature.

Terminology: ''The forehead feels warm and dry.''

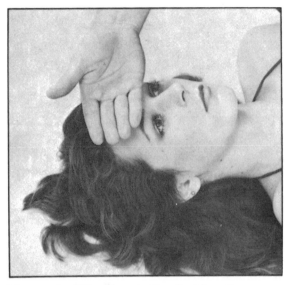

Figure 1–23   Touch the forehead.

3. Eyelids   Check the eyelids for raccoon or owl appearance (Figure 1.24) (discoloration around eyes without local swelling; Figure 1.25).

Terminology: ''The eyelids are not discolored.''

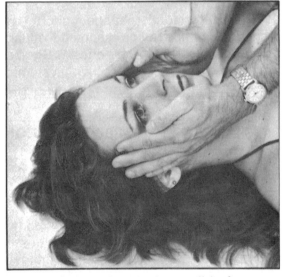

Figure 1–24   Check the eyelids for raccoon eyes.

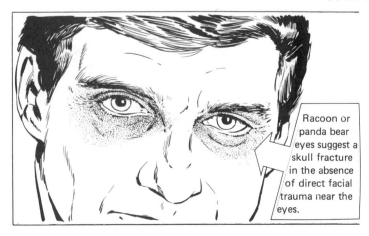

Racoon or panda bear eyes suggest a skull fracture in the absence of direct facial trauma near the eyes.

Figure 1–25

STEP	SPECIFIC MOTION

continued

4. Pupils   Examine the pupils for equality and reaction to light (Figure 1.26).

Terminology: "The pupils are equal and react to light."

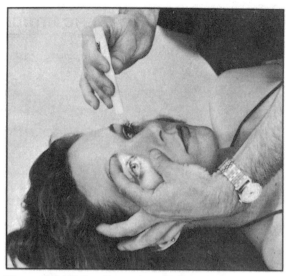

Figure 1–26   Examine the pupils.

5. Conjunctiva   Pull either lower eyelid down to check for color on the inside of the lid—pink or pale (Figure 1.27). Note if eyelids resist opening.

Terminology: "The conjunctiva are pink."

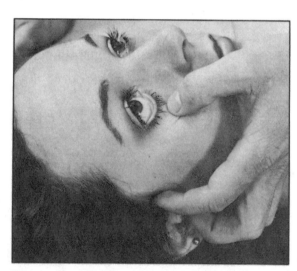

Figure 1–27   Check the conjunctiva color.

STEP	SPECIFIC MOTION

continued

6. Nose

Check the nose for flaring, deformity, bleeding, or leaking of clear fluid (Figure 1.28).

Terminology: ''There is no blood or fluid coming from the nose.''

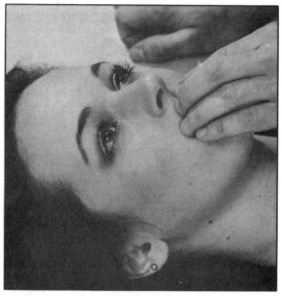

Figure 1–28   Inspect the nose for fluid discharge.

7. Ears

Inspect the ears for blood or clear fluid without turning the patient's head (Figure 1.29).

Terminology: ''There is no blood or fluid coming from the ears.''

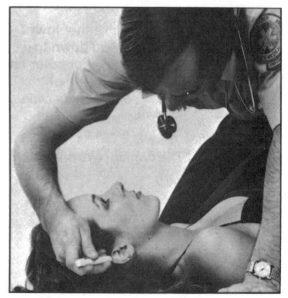

Figure 1–29   Inspect the ears for fluid discharge.

STEP	SPECIFIC MOTION

continued

8. Mastoids

Check over the mastoids for bruising or discoloration (Figures 1.30 to 1.32).

Terminology: ''There are no Battle's signs.''

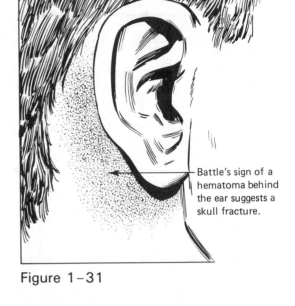

— Battle's sign of a hematoma behind the ear suggests a skull fracture.

Figure 1–31

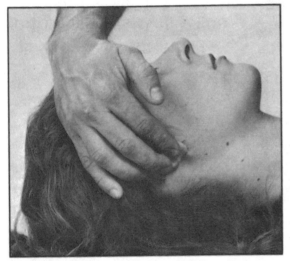

Figure 1–30   Look for Battle's signs.

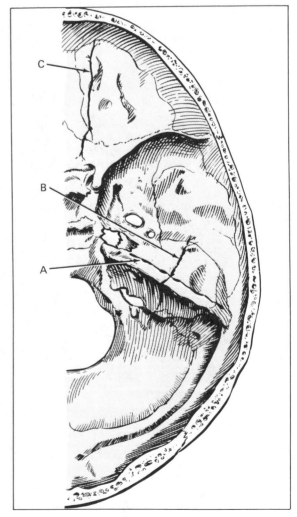

Figure 1–32   Battle's sign basilar skull fracture. Longitudinal (A) and transverse (B) fractures of petrous pyramid of temporal bone and anterior basal skull fracture (C).

STEP	SPECIFIC MOTION

continued

9. Facial bones — Palpate the zygomatic arches and mandible for tenderness (Figures 1.33 and 1.34).

Terminology: "There is no facial bone tenderness."

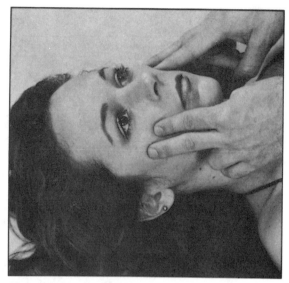

Figure 1–33 Palpate zygoma for fractures.

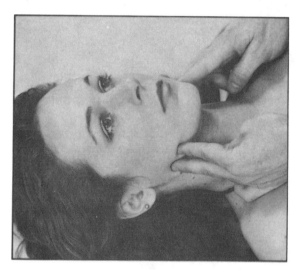

Figure 1–34 Palpate mandible for fractures.

10. Mouth — Examine the mouth for loose teeth, abnormal alignment, and oral hydration (Figure 1.35). Check for perioral cyanosis.

Terminology: "There are no loose teeth, alignment is normal, and oral hydration is normal. There is no perioral cyanosis."

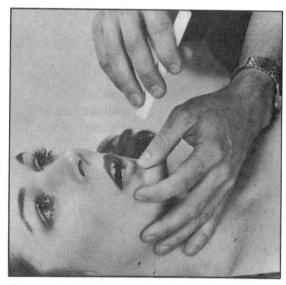

Figure 1–35 Examine the mouth for loose teeth.

STEP	SPECIFIC MOTION

continued

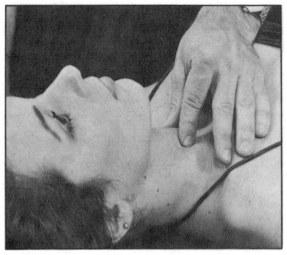

Figure 1-36   Check for tracheal shift.

11. Neck/trachea — Inspect for a midline trachea (Figure 1.36), stoma, and Medicalert necklace.

Terminology: "The trachea is midline with no stoma or Medicalert necklace."

12. Suprasternal area — Check the suprasternal area for retractions, hypertrophy of accessory muscles of respiration (Figure 1.37), or subcutaneous emphysema.

Terminology: "There are no suprasternal retractions, hypertrophy of accessory muscles of respiration, or subcutaneous emphysema."

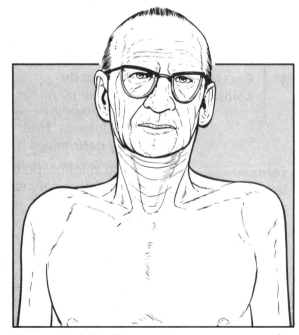

Figure 1-37   Observe accessory muscle size.

STEP	SPECIFIC MOTION

continued

13. Neck veins

Check the neck for neck vein distension. If present, see if the veins fill from above (the head) or below (the heart) (Figure 1.38).

Terminology: "The neck veins show no filling from below except when the patient is supine.

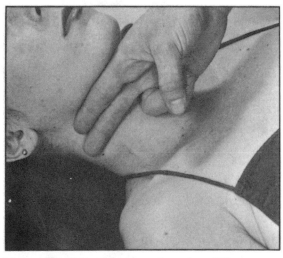

Figure 1–38   Note neck veins filling from below.

14. Cervical spine

Palpate the cervical spine for midline point tenderness (Figure 1.39). Note swelling or any deformity.

Terminology: "There is no midline point tenderness or deformity of the cervical spine."

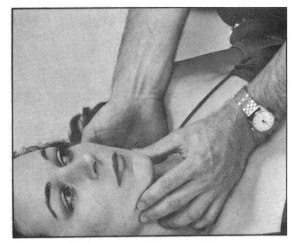

Figure 1–39   Palpate the cervical spine.

15. Chest wall

Observe the chest wall for any area of flailing (paradoxical breathing; Figure 1.40). Note discoloration or any splinting or retractions. Palpate down the sternum.

Terminology: "There is no flail chest wall segment, splinting, or retractions."

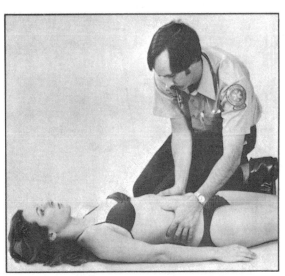

Figure 1–40   Observe for flail chest.

STEP	SPECIFIC MOTION

continued

16. Ribs

Check for any tenderness during chest compression (Figure 1.41). Do not push over any obvious bruise.

Terminology: "There is no tenderness on compression of the ribs."

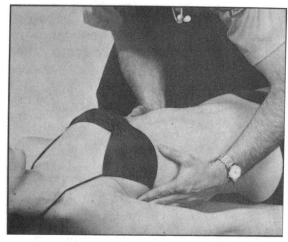

Figure 1–41   Test for rib compression pain.

17. Thoracic spine*

Palpate the thoracic spine as well as possible without rolling the patient (Figure 1.42).

Terminology: "There is no point tenderness of the thoracic spine."

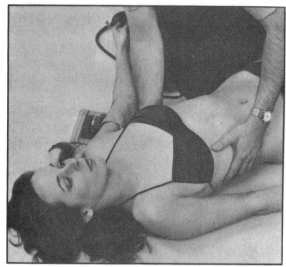

Figure 1–42   Palpate the thoracic spine.

18. Pleural space

Auscultate the chest during inspiration at the anterior axillary line for equal air entry (Figure 1.43).

Terminology: "There is equal air entry into the chest."

*This step is optional since the thoracic spine is hard to feel unless the patient is turned.

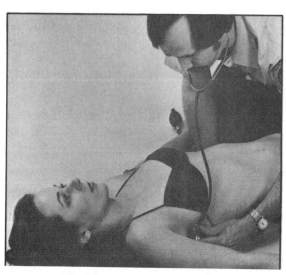

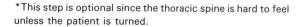

Figure 1–43   Auscultate for equal air entry.

STEP	SPECIFIC MOTION

continued

19. Breath sounds — Auscultate anteriorly and posteriorly to detect the quality of breath sounds (Figure 1.44).

Terminology: "The posterior lung fields reveal no rales or wheezes."

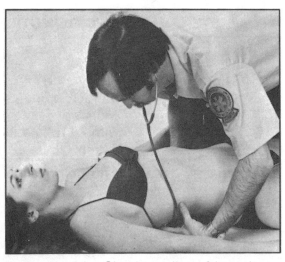

Figure 1–44   Check quality of breath sounds.

20. Heart — Auscultate the heart for apical rate and possibility of muffled heart tones (Figure 1.45).

Terminology: "There is no progressive muffling of the heart tones, no apical pulse deficit, and no cardiac irregularity."

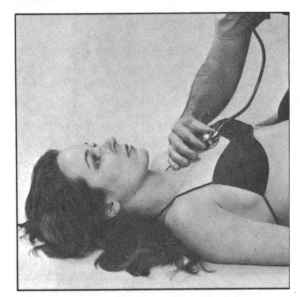

Figure 1–45   Listen for muffled heart tones.

21. Abdominal wall — Observation: Look at the abdomen for distension, wounds, or evisceration of bowel (Figure 1.46).

Terminology: "There is no bowel evisceration."

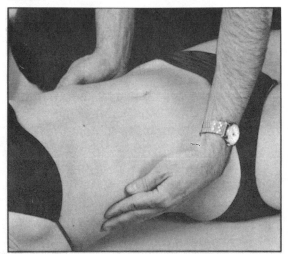

Figure 1–46   Check the abdomen for evisceration.

STEP	SPECIFIC MOTION

continued

22. Bowel sounds

Auscultation: Auscultate the abdomen for bowel sounds (Figure 1.47). If absent, mention the amount of time listening.*

Terminology: "The bowel sounds are normal."

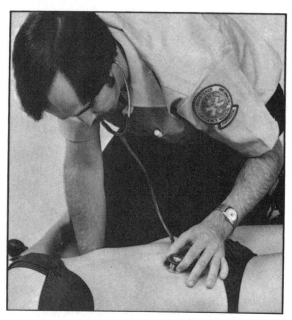

Figure 1–47   Auscultate for bowel sounds.

23. Abdominal tenderness

Palpation: Inspect the abdomen for penetration. Palpate the abdomen in all four quadrants for tenderness (Figure 1.48).

Terminology: "The abdomen is soft, nontender in all four quadrants, without bruises or lacerations."

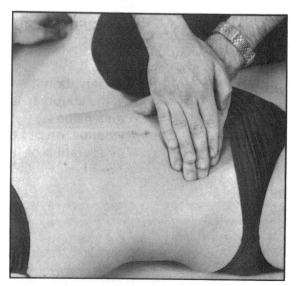

Figure 1–48   Palpate for abdominal tenderness.

*Rarely used in prehospital care—instructor option.

STEP	SPECIFIC MOTION

continued

24. Lumbar spine   Palpate the low back for midline point tenderness (Figure 1.49).

Terminology: "There is no midline point tenderness of the lumbar spine."

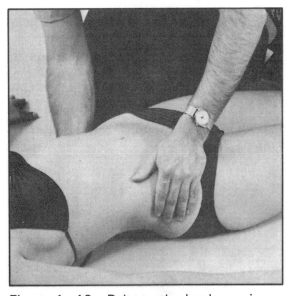

Figure 1–49   Palpate the lumbar spine.

25. Pelvis   Compress the pelvis inward and downward with hands covering the hip joint and iliac crest (Figures 1.50 and 1.51). Note any pubic tenderness or incontinence. (Priapism— persistent erection—if present would be communicated as a sign of possible spinal cord damage.)

Terminology: "There is no tenderness upon pelvic compression and no evidence of incontinence."

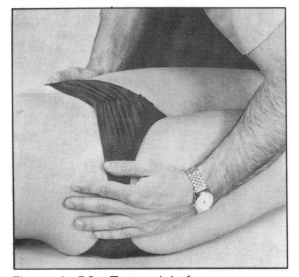

Figure 1–50   Test pelvis for compression pain.

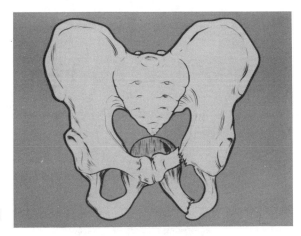

Figure 1–51   Pelvic fracture discovered upon compression of the pelvis.

STEP	SPECIFIC MOTION

continued

26. Legs/femoral pulses*

Palpate the femoral pulses for equality (Figure 1.52).

Terminology: "Femoral pulses are equal and strong."

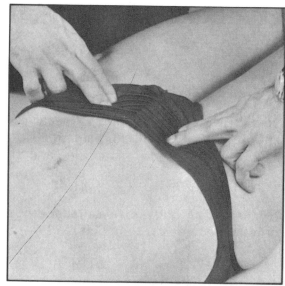

Figure 1–52   Palpate the femoral pulses.

27. Deformity

Inspect and palpate both legs for bleeding, tenderness, and deformity (Figure 1.53).

Terminology: "There is no deformity, laceration, or area of point tenderness in the legs."

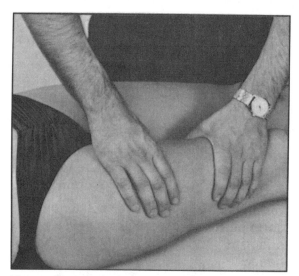

Figure 1–53   Check legs for point tenderness.

28. Calves and tibias

Check the calves for tenderness on squeezing (Figure 1.54), and the tibias for pitting edema (Figure 1.55).

Terminology: "There is no midline calf tenderness or pitting edema over the tibia."

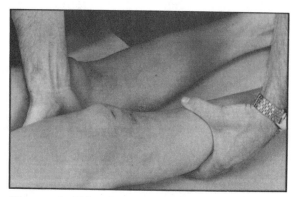

Figure 1–54   Palpate midline calf for tenderness.

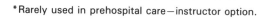

*Rarely used in prehospital care—instructor option.

STEP	SPECIFIC MOTION

continued

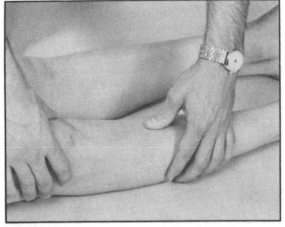

Figure 1–55   Examine the tibia for edema.

29. Pedal pulses

Palpate both feet for either the dorsalis pedis pulse or posterior tibial pulse* (Figures 1.56 to 1.58).

Terminology: ''The pedal pulses are present bilaterally.''

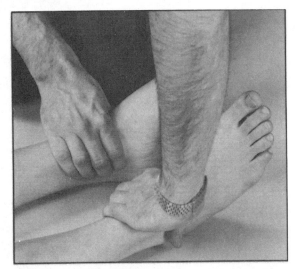

Figure 1–56   Palpate the pedal pulses.

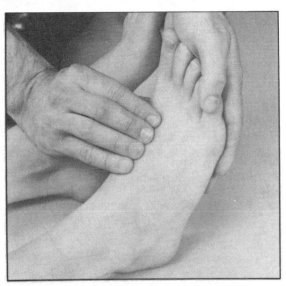

*Either of the pulses shown above may be palpated to complete this step.

Figure 1–57   Dorsalis pedis pulse.

STEP	SPECIFIC MOTION

continued

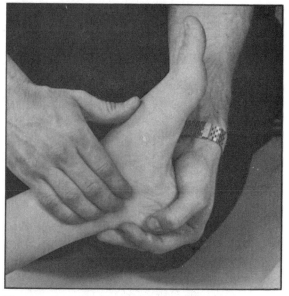

Figure 1-58   Posterior tibial pulse.

30. Foot sensation

Ask patient to determine which toe is touched by the rescuer (Figure 1.59).

Terminology: "Sensation is intact in both feet."

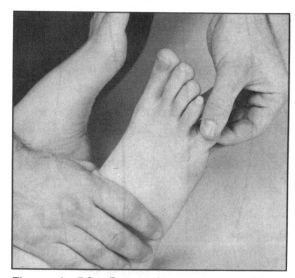

Figure 1-59   Determine toe recognition.

STEP	SPECIFIC MOTION

continued

31. Painful withdrawal

Test withdrawal to pressure on large toe nail bed bases bilaterally (Figure 1.60).

Terminology: "Painful withdrawal to nail pressure is symmetrical."

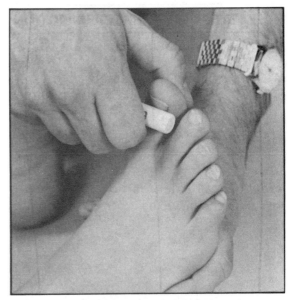

Figure 1–60   Check for withdrawl to pain.

32. Foot movement

Have patient demonstrate ability to wave both feet (Figures 1.61 and 1.62), then check the strength of extension.

Terminology: "Voluntary movement is intact and strength is equal bilaterally in the legs."

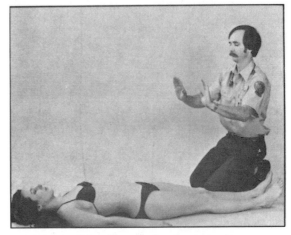

Figure 1–61   Teach foot wave to patient.

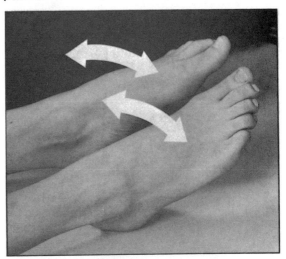

Figure 1–62   Observe foot wave.

STEP	SPECIFIC MOTION

continued

33. Reflexes*   Test knee jerk and ankle jerk reflexes using a reflex hammer (Figures 1.63 and 1.64).

Terminology: "Knee jerks and ankle jerks are equal bilaterally. Babinski reflexes are negative."

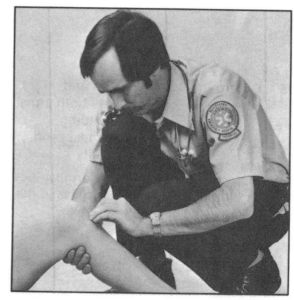

Figure 1-63   Test knee jerk reflexes.

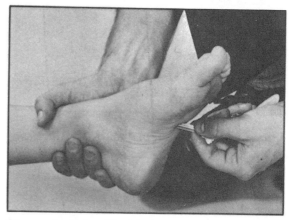

Figure 1-64   Check for Babinski reflexes.

34. Arms/clavicles   Palpate both clavicles from the sternum toward the shoulder for tenderness or deformity (Figure 1.65).

Terminology: "There is no point tenderness over the clavicles."

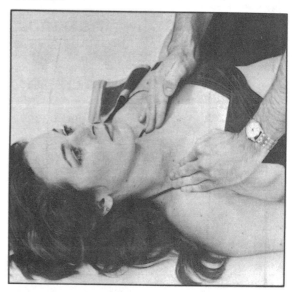

Figure 1-65   Palpate for clavicular fractures.

*Rarely used in prehospital care—instructor option.

STEP	SPECIFIC MOTION

continued

35. Deformity — Inspect and palpate both arms for bleeding, tenderness, and deformity (Figure 1.66).

Terminology: "There is no deformity, laceration, or area of point tenderness in the arms."

36. Radial pulses — Compare radial pulses for presence and equality (Figure 1.67). (If unequal, compare BPs bilaterally).

Terminology: "The radial pulses are present and equal bilaterally."

37. Hand sensation — Ask patient to determine which finger is touched by the rescuer (Figure 1.68).

Terminology: "Sensation is intact in both hands."

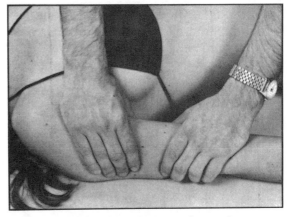

Figure 1–66   Check arms for point tenderness.

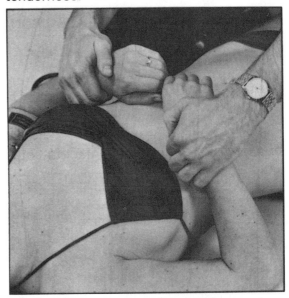

Figure 1–67   Compare radial pulse.

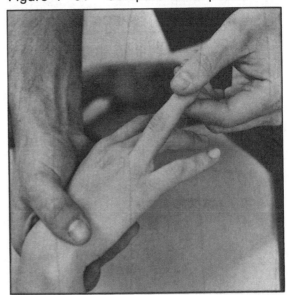

Figure 1–68   Determine finger recognition.

STEP	SPECIFIC MOTION

continued

38. Painful withdrawal

Test withdrawal to pressure on thumb nail bed bases bilaterally (Figure 1.69).

Terminology: ''Painful withdrawal to nail pressure is symmetrical.''

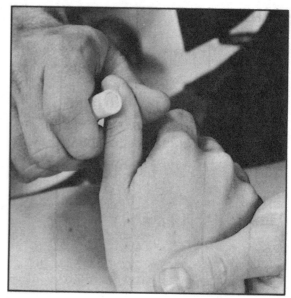

Figure 1–69   Determine withdrawal to pain.

39. Hand movement

Instruct patient to wave both hands to confirm flexion and extension (Figure 1.70). Check grip strength.

Terminology: ''Voluntary movement is intact and grip strength is equal bilaterally in both hands.''

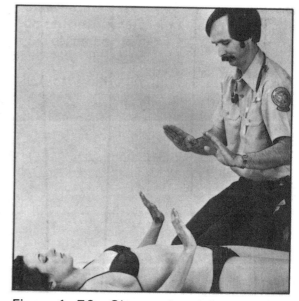

Figure 1–70   Observe hand movement.

STEP	SPECIFIC MOTION

continued

40. Reflexes Test biceps reflexes (Figure 1.71).

Terminology: ''Biceps reflexes are equal bilaterally.''

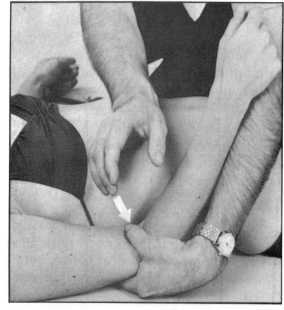

Figure 1–71 Test biceps reflexes.

41. Back—logroll and observe — Logroll the patient, unless spine injury suspected, and observe any posterior wounds (Figure 1.72).

Terminology: ''There are no visible injuries to the back.''

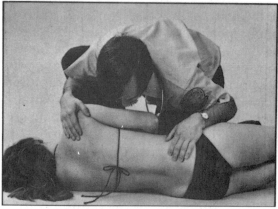

Figure 1–72 Logroll and look at back.

42. Rhythm strip — Check the heart rhythm on the EKG monitor* with leads or paddle readout and get a strip readout. (Figure 1.73).

Terminology: ''The EKG monitor shows normal sinus rhythm.''

This completes the objective exam.

*Covered in Chapter 6.

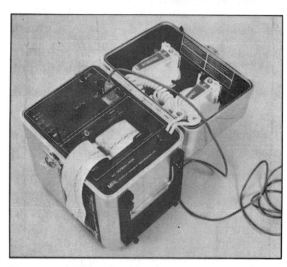

Figure 1–73 Check rhythm on scope and readout.

ASSESSMENT

Although the term *assessment* has various uses, in the SOAP evaluation scheme (Figure 1.74) it stands for the step of drawing a clinical conclusion. In the simplest terms it means "Let's put the subjective and objective information together and decide what's wrong." Common conclusion-type judgments taught at various levels of medical knowledge are listed in Table 1.2. Many physicians feel that if various prehospital rescuers try to make "diagnoses," the word "probable" should be inserted before every conclusion. This can be done where it makes sense, but it would be strange to say "probable ventricular fibrillation," or "probable severely angulated, open fracture of the tibia."

The real issue is that each level of rescuer take the assessment of a patient only to the limits of his or her training. Thus the paramedic can with confidence diagnose an open, angulated fracture of the femur;

PATIENT EVALUATION			
	Life/Death	Critical	Serious
S			
O			
A	A ⟶ G		
P			

Figure 1.74

Table 1.2. JUDGMENTS AT VARIOUS LEVELS OF MEDICAL KNOWLEDGE.

Medical Rescuer	Conclusions	Treatment
Trained citizen	Cafe coronary or foreign body obstruction of the airway	Manual removal
Lifeguard	Cardiac arrest due to drowning	CPR
First responder	Possible cervical spine injury	Cervical immobilization
EMT-Basic	Emergency childbirth with crowning	Prepare to deliver
Paramedic	Hypovolemic shock	Antishock trousers
CCU nurse	Ventricular fibrillation	Defibrillate
Emergency physician	Pericardial tamponade	Pericardiocentesis
Surgeon	Appendicitis	Appendectomy

may wish simply to categorize shock with "hypovolemic shock—possible ruptured spleen," and may show greatest restraint with nontraumatic abdominal pain by saying "peritonitis—cause unclear."

Many times physicians are puzzled about patient conditions and have no reservation about using such broad conclusions as "chest pain—cause unclear" or dyspnea—cause unclear." Another approach used by physicians for hospitalized patients is to admit the patient to exclude a severe problem. Then the diagnosis will read "Chest pain R/O MI" (rule out myocardial infarction).

Table 1.3 shows examples of specific clinical correlations which are often used in assessment of the trauma patient. Assessments usually are developed from at least *three subjective and/or objective criteria;* for example, hypotension, distended neck veins, and muffled heart tones suggest pericardial tamponade.

The *best* assessments of all include not only the problem discovered but the priority threatened. Examples of this approach would be:

1. Probable anaphylaxis but with no laryngoedema

2. Multifocal PVCs with risk of ventricular fibrillation

3. Possible cervical spine fracture with threat to the cervical cord

4. Possible myocardial infarction with risk of dysrhythmia

5. Probable spontaneous pneumothorax without signs of tension

6. Laceration of the right wrist but no evidence of nerve, vessel, or tendon injury

Although such assessments are too long for radio presentations, they are important to stress during training because they help remind the paramedic of the risk of the condition.

Table 1.3. TRAUMA EXAM.

Finding	Possible Correlation
Low BP, high pulse rate	Hypovolemic shock
Low BP, slow pulse rate	Spinal shock
High BP, low pulse rate	Increased intracranial pressure
Raccoon eyes	Basilar skull fracture
Battle's sign	Basilar skull fracture
Clear fluid or blood from ear	Basilar skull fracture
Missing tooth	Aspirated tooth
Subcutaneous air in neck	Ruptured larynx
Point tenderness of cervical spine	Cervical spine fracture
Floating chest segment	Flail chest
Unequal air entry	Hemothorax or pneumothorax
Chest compression pain	Rib fracture
Bowel protrusion through wound	Bowel evisceration
Point tenderness of the lumbar spine	Lumbar spine fracture
Pelvic compression pain	Anterior—bladder injury; posterior—pelvic fracture with hidden blood loss
Tenderness, deformity and grating—extremity	Fracture
Absent pulse in an injured limb	Limb ischemia

A common but even more complicated example would be a fractured jaw. By itself the injury has little meaning in the field. But when one considers the importance of the jaw to the airway and the fact that any jaw trauma means that the brain and neck were subjected to the same force, the priorities become clear. A student demonstrates this level of understanding by observing "a probable fractured mandible but with no compromise of the airway, signs of change in responsiveness, or tenderness of the cervical spine." Such assessments should be encouraged in almost all settings except on the air (radio traffic must be kept to a minimum).

Finally, given multiple injuries, the injury associated with the highest priority is treated first. Using the A-to-G system discussed earlier, a patient with fractured femur, pneumothorax, tracheal injury, and arm abrasion would be assessed in this order:

Probable tracheal injury (A priority)

Possible pneumothorax (B priority)

Fractured femur (C priority*)

Arm abrasion (E priority)

*C priority due to risk of bleeding with this fracture.

Using such an order helps organize a treatment plan and demonstrates priority judgment.

On the Detailed Patient Evaluation Guide the step of assessment is outlined as follows:

ASSESSMENT Conclusion "The probable condition is _____ ."

Priority "The priority threatened is _____ ."

PLAN

The treatment plan comes directly from the assessment and should also follow the A-to-G scheme (Figure 1.75). The paramedic is required to do noninvasive EMT-Basic skills before calling in to the hospital. Therefore, the usual sequence is to tell the hospital what EMT-Basic skills have been done and then ask for permission to do advanced skills. This is the way the Guide is set up.

Naturally, when there are many standing orders, the paramedic can solve problems such as airway obstruction at both levels immediately:

• Lift the jaw (basic).

• Intubate (advanced).

PATIENT EVALUATION			
	Life/Death	Critical	Serious
S	Chief complaint	History of present illness	Past medical history Meds Allergies
O	Primary survey A ⟶ D	Intermediate survey A ⟶ D	Secondary survey Head ⟶ Toe
A	A ⟶ G		
P	A ⟶ G		

Figure 1.75

The important principle is to lay out the plan in the same A-to-G sequence as the assessment.

Finally, a plan must include transportation. The three final elements are transportation code, patient position, and ETA (estimated time of arrival). *Remember that the ETA being reported on the radio should* include *loading and transport time.*

The transportation code should be rapid (Code 3—lights and siren) only if the patient's condition warrants it and if the sound and movement will not cause further deterioration of the patient. The patient's position should be thought about prior to loading, including whether you want to put your patient in feet first, as perhaps with tall patients with traction splints.

LAB PRACTICE

The following Detailed Patient Evaluation Guide is to be used during lab practice of this skill. Paired students take turns being rescuer and evaluator.

DETAILED PATIENT EVALUATION GUIDE

Rescuer's Name_____ Date_____ Evaluator_____

Directions for Evaluator: Place a check beside each item whenever an exam is omitted, performed improperly, or presented improperly.

Sample Patient Problem: 55-year-old male develops chest pain while driving and crashes into an oak tree. Has mild concussion. Rescue coordinator present.

Exam Step	Memory Aid	Question or Presentation	Question Asked	Presentation of Information
SUBJECTIVE				
A. Interview rescue coordinator (if available)	Overview	What happened?	_____	_____
	Position	Was he a driver or passenger?	_____	_____
	Blood loss	Any external blood loss?	_____	_____
	Responsiveness	Was he briefly awake after the accident before passing out?	_____	_____
	Mechanism of injury	How fast was he going? Was he thrown from the car?	_____	_____
B. Interview of patient				
1. Introduction and reassurance		I am paramedic Dave Williams. May I help you? What is your name?	_____	_____
2. Chief complaint		What is your main problem?	_____	_____
3. History of present illness	Provocation	What brought it on?	_____	_____
	Quality	What does it feel like?	_____	_____

DETAILED PATIENT EVALUATION GUIDE, continued

Exam Step	Memory Aid	Question or Presentation	Question Asked	Presentation of Information
	Radiation	Where else does it go?	_____	_____
	Severity	How bad is it?	_____	_____
	Time	How long has it lasted?	_____	_____
4. Age		How old are you?	_____	_____
5. Past medical health a. Illnesses		Are you under a doctor's care for anything?	_____	_____
b. Current medications		Do you take any prescription drugs?	_____	_____
c. Allergies		Are you allergic to any drugs?	_____	_____

OBJECTIVE

A. Primary survey	1. Airway	Respirations are quiet.	_____	_____
	2. Breathing	Breathing is unlabored.	_____	_____
	3. Circulation	The skin is pink with no external bleeding.	_____	_____
	4. Delicate CNS	Patient responds to voice and moves all four limbs easily.	_____	_____
B. Vital signs	1. Respiration	The respirations are normal in depth and effort.	_____	_____
	2. Pulse	The pulse is strong and regular.	_____	_____

DETAILED PATIENT EVALUATION GUIDE, continued

Exam Step	Memory Aid	Question or Presentation	Question Asked	Presentation of Information
	3. Palpable BP	The palpable BP is _____	_____	_____
	4. Full BP	The full BP is _____	_____	_____
C. Secondary survey (head to toe)	1. Scalp	The scalp is not bleeding and the skull shows no deformity.	_____	_____
1. Head	2. Forehead	The forehead feels warm and dry.	_____	_____
	3. Eyelids	The eyelids are not discolored.	_____	_____
	4. Pupils	The pupils are equal and react to light.	_____	_____
	5. Conjunctiva	The conjunctiva are pink.	_____	_____
	6. Nose	There is no blood or fluid coming from the nose.	_____	_____
	7. Ears	There is no blood or fluid coming from the ears.	_____	_____
	8. Mastoids	There are no Battle's signs.	_____	_____
	9. Facial bones	There is no facial bone tenderness.	_____	_____
	10. Mouth	There are no loose teeth, alignment is normal, and oral hydration is normal. There is no perioral cyanosis.	_____	_____

DETAILED PATIENT EVALUATION GUIDE, continued

Exam Step	Memory Aid	Question or Presentation	Question Asked	Presentation of Information
2. Neck	1. Trachea	The trachea is midline with no stoma or Medicalert necklace.	_____	_____
	2. Suprasternal area	There are no suprasternal retractions, hypertrophy of accessory muscles of respiration, or subcutaneous emphysema.	_____	_____
	3. Neck veins	The neck veins show no filling from below except when the patient is supine.	_____	_____
	4. Cervical spine	There is no midline point tenderness or deformity of the cervical spine.	_____	_____
3. Chest	1. Chest wall	There is no flail chest wall segment, splinting, or retractions.	_____	_____
	2. Ribs	There is no tenderness on compression of the chest wall.	_____	_____
	3. Thoracic spine	There is no point tenderness of the thoracic spine.	_____	_____
	4. Pleural space	There is equal air entry into the chest.	_____	_____

DETAILED PATIENT EVALUATION GUIDE, continued

Exam Step	Memory Aid	Question or Presentation	Question Asked	Presentation of Information
	5. Breath sounds	The posterior lung fields reveal no rales or wheezes.	_____	_____
	6. Heart	There is no progressive muffling of the heart tones, no apical pulse deficit, and no cardiac irregularity.	_____	_____
4. Abdomen	1. Observation	There is no bowel evisceration.	_____	_____
	2. Auscultation	The bowel sounds are normal.	_____	_____
	3. Palpation	The abdomen is soft, nontender in all four quadrants, without bruises or lacerations.	_____	_____
5. Lumbar spine	1. Palpate	There is no midline point tenderness of the lumbar spine.	_____	_____
6. Pelvis	1. Compress	There is no tenderness upon pelvic compression and no evidence of incontinence.	_____	_____
7. Legs	1. Femoral pulses	Femoral pulses are equal and strong.	_____	_____

DETAILED PATIENT EVALUATION GUIDE, continued

Exam Step	Memory Aid	Question or Presentation	Question Asked	Presentation of Information
	2. Deformity	There is no deformity, laceration, or area of point tenderness in the legs.	_____	_____
	3. Calves and tibias	There is no calf tenderness nor pitting edema over the tibia.	_____	_____
	4. Pedal pulses	The pedal pulses are present bilaterally.	_____	_____
	5. Foot sensation	Sensation is intact in both feet.	_____	_____
	6. Painful withdrawal	Painful withdrawal to nail pressure is symmetrical.	_____	_____
	7. Foot movement	Voluntary movement is intact and strength is equal bilaterally in the legs.	_____	_____
	8. Reflexes	Knee jerks and ankle jerks are equal bilaterally. Babinski reflexes are negative.	_____	_____
8. Arms	1. Clavicles	There is no point tenderness over the clavicles.	_____	_____
	2. Deformity	There is no deformity, laceration, or area of point tenderness in the arms.	_____	_____

DETAILED PATIENT EVALUATION GUIDE, continued

Exam Step	Memory Aid	Question or Presentation	Question Asked	Presentation of Information
	3. Radial pulses	The radial pulses are present and equal bilaterally.	_____	_____
	4. Hand sensation	Sensation is intact in both hands.	_____	_____
	5. Painful withdrawal	Painful withdrawal to nail pressure is symmetrical.	_____	_____
	6. Hand movement	Voluntary movement is intact and grip strength is equal bilaterally in both hands.	_____	_____
	7. Reflexes	Biceps and triceps reflexes are equal bilaterally.	_____	_____
9. Back	1. Logroll and observation	There are no visible injuries to the back.	_____	_____
10. Rhythm	1. Rhythm by scope	The EKG monitor shows normal sinus rhythm.	_____	_____

ASSESSMENT

	Conclusion	1. The probable condition is ____	_____	_____
	Priority	2. The priority threatened is ____	_____	_____

DETAILED PATIENT EVALUATION GUIDE, continued

Exam Step	Memory Aid	Question or Presentation	Question Asked	Presentation of Information
PLAN				
	Paramedic	1. Airway— ___		_____
	A to G	2. Breathing—		_____
		3. Circulation—		_____
		4. Delicate CNS— _____		_____
		5. External soft tissue—		_____
		6. Fracture—		_____
		7. GI/GU—		_____
	Code	1. The patient will be transported Code		_____
	Position	2. In _____ position.		_____
	ETA	3. Our ETA is		_____

Note: Rescuer gets credit on this part of the plan if the skills are appropriate and basically in the order noted here. Where there is no skill in a certain priority, nothing need be mentioned.

SUMMARY

A good patient examination is a process that discovers conditions rather than assuming them. The paramedic is a physician extender and must gather information for the physician with thoroughness, speed, and precision. The exam is first learned as a long and exacting procedure with the patient supine and cooperative. This allows practice of good technique and good verbalization. Later the patient exam is made more difficult by changing the patient condition and body positions and by adding distracting factors such as noise. Once the student has this solid foundation, he or she can begin to take shortcuts. To avoid letting shortcuts become bad habits, the full exam must be repracticed monthly and become the foundation of any refresher program.

SKILL PROFICIENCY TESTING

Skill Advanced Patient Examination

Performance Demonstrate how to complete an advanced-level patient examination, relaying what you are doing during the examination and then orally relaying the assessment and plan to a second rescuer.

Conditions

1. Simulated 55-year-old male who developed pain while driving and has crashed into a tree. Had mild concussion with transient confusion now resolving.*

2. Patient positioned face up on blanket, in moderate but not severe distress. Patient is able to answer questions.

3. Evaluator first simulates a first-in responder who has the sign "Rescue Coordinator" on chest.

4. After the oral interview, evaluator will turn the sign over with the label "Fellow Rescuer" showing. This will remind the rescuer to direct comments about exam, assessment, and plan to this person.

5. Equipment—blood pressure cuff, stethoscope, penlight, scratch pad, and pencil next to patient on blanket.

6. Rescuer sits outside testing room reading above information. When the room is ready, he is told to come in and start.

Standard

1. Rescuer examines patient according to the contents and general SOAP sequence of the Detailed Patient Examination Guide. ☐

2. Objective findings both normal and abnormal, the assessment, and the plan are relayed to the evaluator as they are done. ☐

3. Terminology follows that used in the same guide. ☐

4. Entire examination is completed without omitting more than four exam steps. ☐

5. Examination with presentation is completed within 7 minutes. ☐

Student's Name_____ Date_____ Evaluator_____

Pass/Fail

*Note: This type of patient is encouraged because the problem involves a medical problem (chest pain), trauma problem (steering wheel injury), and neural problem (concussion).

2

Airway Skills

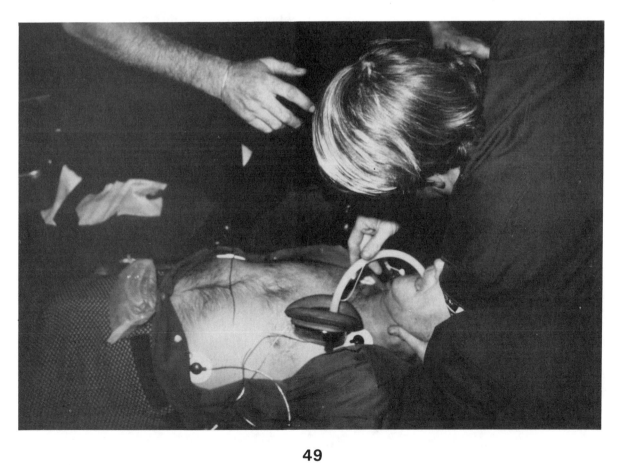

Skills Objectives

- **Esophageal Obturator Airway Insertion**—Demonstrate how to prepare, insert, test, secure, and later remove an esophageal obturator airway using an adult intubation manikin.

- **Adult Endotracheal Intubation**—Demonstrate how to prepare, insert, test, secure, and later remove a No. 8 orral endotracheal tube in an adult intubation manikin.

- **Infant Endotracheal Intubation**—Demonstrate how to prepare, insert, test, secure, and later remove a No. 3 endotracheal tube in an infant intubation manikin.

- **Endotracheal Suctioning**—Demonstrate how to suction mucus properly from a patient with a secured endotracheal tube.

- **Percutaneous Cricothyrotomy**—(extraordinary) Demonstrate how to perform a cricothyrotomy on an anesthetized dog or suitable manikin using a Nu-Trach or Pedia-Trach predesigned kit.

- **Surgical Cricothyrotomy**—(extraordinary) Demonstrate how to perform a cricothyrotomy on an anesthetized dog or suitable manikin.

Outline

Airway Skills Description

Esophageal Obturator Airway Insertion
Adult Endotracheal Intubation
Infant Endotracheal Intubation
Endotracheal Suctioning
Percutaneous Cricothyrotomy
Surgical Cricothyrotomy

Skill Proficiency Testing

Introduction
Special Considerations

Judgment
Equipment
Skill Sequence
Lab Practice

Airway Skills Description

INTRODUCTION

Airway refers to the passageway to the lungs; *breathing* involves the mechanics of moving air in and out of the lungs. Rather than combining these two critical areas into the heading "respiration," this book has sought separation so that the rescuer will approach each step in the ABCs independently and in order. Rescuers at all levels, from citizens at the scene to the emergency physician, must make obtaining and maintaining an open airway the first patient treatment priority in any condition!

There are many airway skills taught at the EMT-Basic level, including jaw lifts, neck hyperextension, suctioning, coma body positioning (see Figures 2.1 and 2.2), and maneuvers for removing meat, food, or other objects caught in the pharynx. The advanced rescuers must have a mastery of these skills but must also know when to apply more invasive skills, such as the use of the endotracheal tube, esophageal obturator airway, and endotracheal suctioning. Many physicians teach paramedics to perform needle cricothyrotomy or surgical cricothyrotomy to establish an airway or to allow oxygen insufflation.

The art of handling these advanced skills involves not only mastering the techniques but also learning when to stay within the basic EMT skills. Many times a patient whose airway is compromised in the supine position but who is only mildly sedated will be better handled in the side (lateral recumbent) position than with an attempt at intubation. If the advanced airway techniques are generally reserved for patients with progressive cyanosis, deep unresponsiveness with shallow respiration, or full cardiac arrest, they can be truly useful and lifesaving.

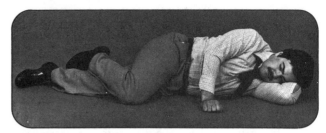

Figure 2–1   Left lateral.

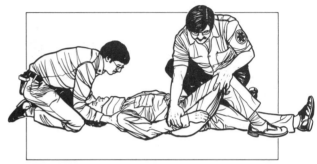

Figure 2–2   Turning the unconscious trauma patient (used if vomiting anticipated or starting to occur).

SPECIAL CONSIDERATIONS

For all mammals, the vital airway passage is connected through the pharynx with the digestive system; medical rescue would be much simpler if this were not true. However, paramedics and other rescuers must deal daily with complications of this connection, such as relaxation of the patient's tongue back into the pharynx, cafe coronary, vomiting with aspiration, and traumatic disruption of the mouth, nose, and trachea.

Airway skills are designed to establish a clear pathway for respiration. Basic skills deal mainly with secretions and the tongue: oropharyngeal airway, coma position, removing vomitus, and so on. Advanced skills are designed to prevent vomiting with aspiration, directly seal the airway, or create a new airway.

Esophageal Obturator Airway Insertion

The esophageal obturator airway (EOA) was designed both to hold the tongue away from the pharynx and to allow positive pressure ventilation, while preventing air from going into the stomach and gastric acid coming back into the pharynx. Its principal advantage over an endotracheal (ET) tube is its easy placement with minimal training. Its main disadvantages are that it does not allow a direct pathway into the larynx for suctioning, it depends on a good mask face seal for ventilation, and hyperextension of the neck after insertion. When both the EOA and ET tubes are available, the ET tube is generally preferred.

JUDGMENT

Indications

The esophageal obturator airway is indicated for deeply unconscious patients with shallow respiration, progressive cyanosis, and cardiopulmonary arrest.

Contraindications

The esophageal obturator airway is contraindicated in a patient with a gag reflex, a patient under age 16, a patient with facial damage where the mask cannot seal properly; a patient with esophageal disease, as in cirrosis of the liver with varices; and a patient who may wake up with naloxone (Narcan) or 50% dextrose.

Precautions

The rescuer must remove the tube either with an awakening patient on his or her side or with a patient in persisting coma after replacement with an endotracheal tube. Have suction equipment ready in either case.

Complication

Esophageal tears have occurred. Inadvertent tracheal placement must be recognized immediately and the tube removed.

EQUIPMENT

The equipment includes the obturator tube (Figure 2.3), the mask, a 35-ml syringe, and a package of water-base lubricant. The entire kit can be held together with a rubber band and be quite handy. An alternative tube has been developed to allow gastric suctioning (EGTA) and is pictured (Figure 2.4) for comparison. Note that the latter has no side holes, and air must be put in the correct hole.

Many areas prefer EGTA because of the suctioning ability. Both tubes must be used

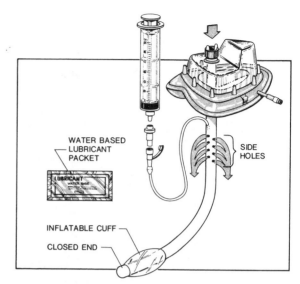

Figure 2–3   Esophageal Obturator Airway (EOA).

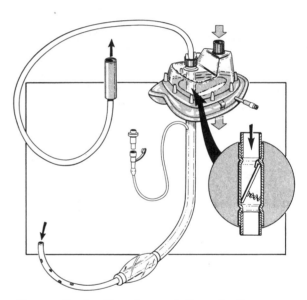

Figure 2–4   Esophageal Gastric Tube Airway (EGTA).

with increased caution in hot climates because of increased flexibility and kinking.

SKILL SEQUENCE

The following skill sequence integrates the use of the esophageal airway during CPR (see Figures 2.5 to 2.8).

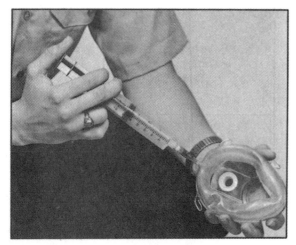

Figure 2–5   Inflate mask.

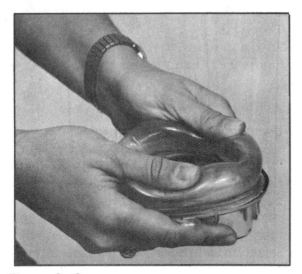

Figure 2–6

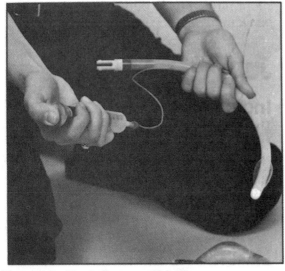

Figure 2–7   Inflate cuff balloon.

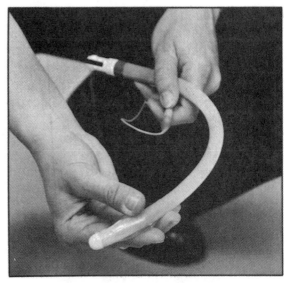

Figure 2–8   Test cuff balloon.

Check the Equipment

The rescuer first checks to make sure that the mask, tube, syringe, and lubricant packet are all present. If an oil-base lubricant has gotten into the kit, it should be replaced by a water-base lubricant. Next the balloon is tested by inflating with 35 ml of air. Once tested, the cuff is deflated in preparation for insertion. The foregoing steps can be done during the morning ambulance check-off to help expedite placement during the rescue call. Then the mask is filled with air and placed over the tube, oriented for placement over the face. Lubricant may be placed on the tip of the tube.

Use the Proper Grip

The rescuer generally uses the left hand to grasp the patient's jaw and inserts the esophageal obturator airway using the right hand. The tube is grasped just below the mask.

Interrupt CPR

After four rapid ventilations, you do not need to stop chest compressions for EOA insertion, CPR is interrupted and the patient's neck is returned to neutral position.

Insert the Tube

In the nontrauma patient, the rescuer slightly flexes the neck and lifts up on the mandible with left thumb and index finger without hyperextending the neck; the tube is inserted following the curve of the pharynx until the mask settles on the face (Figures 2.9 to 2.11). Hard pushing is not needed or allowed. A pencil grip on the EOA ensures delicate handling.

Seal the Face and Test the Placement

The rescuer lifts up the mandible to accomplish a good two-handed face mask seal (Figure 2.12). Then the rescuer blows into

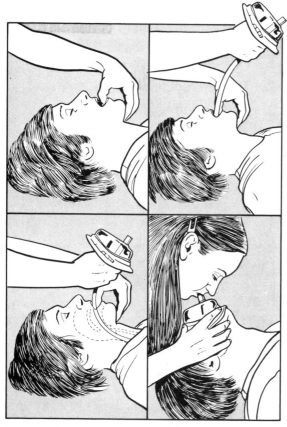

Figure 2–9   Overview of insertion of esophageal obturator airway.

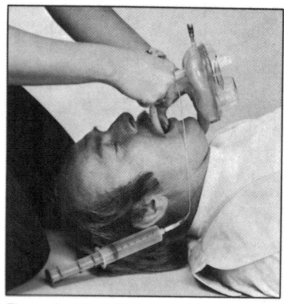

Figure 2–11   Mid-insertion.

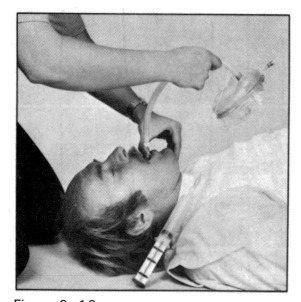

Figure 2–10

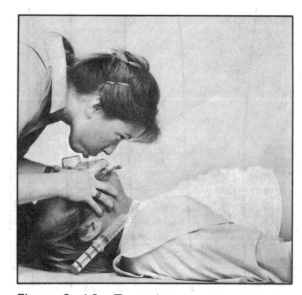

Figure 2–12   Test placement.

the tube for a ventilation if alone, or an assistant ventilates with a big mask or other positive-pressure device. He or she watches to see that the chest expands. If not, the tube must quickly be removed.

Inflate the Balloon

The rescuer next puts 35 ml of air into the syringe adapter to inflate the balloon (Figure 2.13). The syringe must then be removed

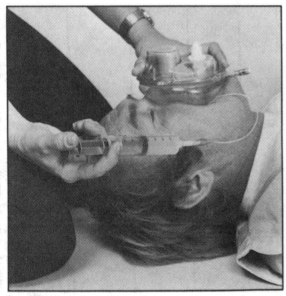

Figure 2–13　Inflate balloon.

to allow the self-sealing valve to keep the air in the balloon.

Listen to the Chest

Use both hands to lift the mandible up to the mask. This time, listen to both sides of the chest with inflation (Figure 2.14).

Ventilate

Using a bag–valve–mask per new JAMA, the rescuer should ventilate once every 5 seconds according to CPR protocol.

Remove the EOA

The rescuer should be able to explain that proper removal consists either of prior replacement with an endotracheal tube in an unconscious patient, or, in a conscious patient, removal with the patient on the side.

1.　Pop off face mask.

2.　Turn patient to side.

3.　Have suction on and readily available.

4.　Deflate cuff balloon (Figure 2.15).

(continues on page 57)

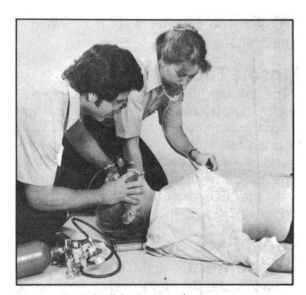

Figure 2–14　Listen to chest.

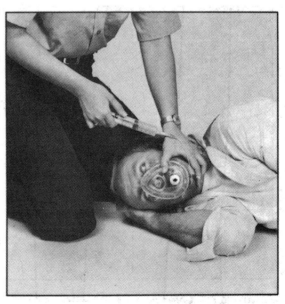

Figure 2–15　Deflate balloon.

ESOPHAGEAL AIRWAY PROCEDURE GUIDE

Rescuer's Name_____ Date_____ Evaluator_____

Directions for Evaluator: Place a check beside each item whenever an exam step is omitted, performed improperly, or presented improperly.

Step	Method	Evaluation
1. Check the equipment	a. Check for presence of mask, obturator tube, 35-ml syringe, lubricant.	_____
	b. Test cuff balloon and then deflate.	_____
	c. Place mask on tube; lubricate obturator tip.*	_____
2. Use the proper grip	a. Grasp tube with right hand below mask.	_____
3. Interrupt vent	a. Tell the rescue crew to stop vent for 15 seconds or less.	_____
4. Insert the tube	a. Return neck to neutral or slightly flexed position.	_____
	b. Lift jaw with left hand.	_____
	c. Insert tube following curve of pharynx until mask is seated on face.	_____
5. Seal the face and test	a. Seal face mask on face using both hands.	_____
	b. Hyperextend neck if no spinal injuries.	_____
	c. Blow in tube and watch chest rise.	_____
6. Resume vent	a. Resume ventilations per tube.	_____
	b. Time limit for stopping CPR less than 15 seconds.	_____
7. Inflate the balloon	a. Inflate cuff balloon with 35 ml of air.	_____
	b. Remove syringe from sealing valve.	_____
8. Listen to the chest	a. Listen to both sides of the chest for equal air entry during ventilation.	_____
9. Ventilate	a. Using a bag–valve–mask, ventilate once every 5 seconds.	_____
10. Remove	a. Pop off face mask.	_____
	b. Turn patient onto side. Have suction on and readily aviable.	_____
	c. Deflate cuff balloon.	_____
	d. Remove following curve of pharynx.	_____
	e. Scoop out any vomitus to clear airway. Suction if necessary.	_____
	f. Keep airway open with jaw maneuvers.	_____

*Do not actually apply to tube since it will harm the manikin.

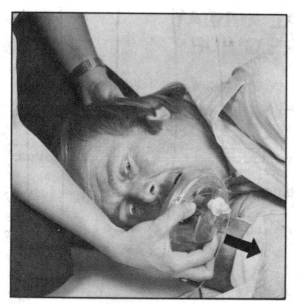

Figure 2–16 Withdraw airway.

5. Remove following curve of pharynx (Figure 2.16).

6. Scoop out any vomitus to clear airway and utilize suction as necessary.

7. Keep airway open with jaw maneuvers.

These steps are summarized in the Esophageal Airway Procedure Guide.

LAB PRACTICE

The preceding Esophageal Airway Procedure Guide is to be used during lab practice of this skill on an intubation manikin. Paired students take turns being rescuer and evaluator.

Adult Endotracheal Intubation

Endotracheal intubation involves direct visualization of the larynx and placement of a tube into the trachea. In the adult the airway is sealed using a balloon, whereas in the infant the trachea narrows below the vocal cords and the tube fits snugly. While the endotracheal (ET) tube may be passed through the nose and into the trachea, it is best learned and performed through the mouth in the emergency prehospital situation.

JUDGMENT

Indications

Endotracheal intubation is indicated for an unconscious patient with shallow respirations, progressive cyanosis, respiratory arrest, and cardiopulmonary arrest. It is also indicated for suctioning in the unconscious patient where mucus or aspiration of vomitus is critically impairing airway.

Contraindications

Enotracheal intubation is contraindicated in a patient with a gag reflex or in a patient ventilating adequately in the left lateral position.

Precautions

The endotracheal balloon and laryngoscope light must be functioning and should be pretested. As with EOA, test equipment at change of shift. The test for proper placement is seeing the chest rise upon ventilation and confirming equal air entry into both lungs by listening with a stethoscope. If possible, do not move the neck when a cervical spine injury is suspected. Attempt placement for maximum of 30 seconds.

Complications

The following complications may occur as a result of endotracheal intubation:

1. Procedure may interrupt CPR for more than 30 seconds.

2. Teeth or dentures may be broken.

3. The tube may be placed in the esophagus or too far down the bronchial tree (into the right mainstem bronchus).

4. Damage to the larynx may occur. This is rare if the ET tube is mandled with a pencil grip and if the stylette does not protrude past the end.

EQUIPMENT

Components of the adult endotracheal intubation kit or tray are (Figure 2.17):

1. No. 8 precut oral ET tube

2. Larynogoscope with No. 4 curved blade

3. No. 4 straight blade

4. 10-ml syringe

5. Kelly clamp unless the cuff balloon has a self-sealing valve

6. Magill forceps

7. Stylet that has been bent at proper length

8. Oral bite block or correct-size OPA

9. Benzoin/adhesive tape or other tube-securing device.

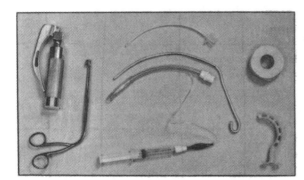

Figure 2–17 Endotracheal intubation kit.

Endotracheal (ET) Tube

An endotracheal tube is a curved tube with a 15-mm adapter at the top and a beveled open end at the bottom, or it has a cuff for sealing connected to an inflation valve. Often, 5 to 10 ml fills the cuff sufficiently.

Overinflation causes damage to the trachea if left for several hours. Either a soft cuff should be used or a little leak allowed if the tube is to stay down very long.

A common problem with endotracheal intubation is insertion of the tube too far, which invariable means that it ends up in the right mainstem bronchus and produces ventilation of only one lung. This occurs because most of the ET tubes on the market are long enough to go through the nose and into the trachea. To prevent overinsertion, these tubes can be precut to a proper oral length. Several companies now produce precut tubes, which saves possible contamination during cutting (Figure 2.18).

Many emergency departments have a No. 7, No. $7\frac{1}{2}$ and a No. 8 endotracheal tube available. Other sizes can be packaged nicely in a wrapped cloth kit that can be unrolled, displaying all sizes.

For long-term ventilation, especially, soft balloon cuffs are used. One design, called "extracorporeal," allows the soft cuff to change size automatically with changes in the trachea. Infant ET tubes have no balloons.

In the child the ET tube size may be guessed from the size of the index finger of the patient. Suction catheters of proper size should be available. Table 2.1 suggests appropriate sizes.

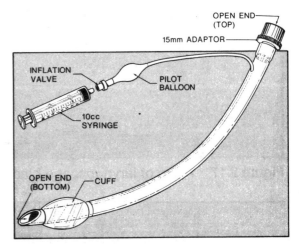

Figure 2–18 Precut (oral) endotracheal tube.

Table 2.1. RECOMMENDED SIZES FOR EN-DOTRACHEAL TUBES AND SUCTION CATHETERS*

Age	Endotracheal Tube Size (Internal Diameter)	Suction Catheters
Newborn	3.0 mm	6 French
6 months	3.5 mm	8 French
18 months	4.0 mm	8 French
3 years	4.5 mm	8 French
5 years	5.0 mm	10 French
6 years	5.5 mm	10 French
8 years	6.0 mm	10 French
12 years	6.5 mm	10 French
16 years	7.0 mm	10 French
Adult (female)	8.0–8.5 mm	12 French
Adult (male)	8.5–9.0 mm	14 French

Source: "Standards for CPR and ECC," *JAMA,* Vol. 227, No. 7, February 18, 1974, p. 854.

*One size larger and one size smaller should be allowed for individual variations.

Just prior to vocal cord visualization, open the sealed package, check the balloon, and replace in the package until ready to insert. Water-soluble lubrication is optional.

Laryngoscope Blades

There are two major types of laryngoscope blades—curved and straight (Figure 2.19). Figure 2.20 shows a side view of the larynx. The epiglottis may be used as a landmark for the curved larynoscope blade (Figure 2.21). In contrast, the epiglottis is lifted up when using a straight blade (Figure 2.22).

The curved blade is the most popular for adult intubation. For pediatric intubation in which the appropriate largyngoscope blade might be harder to choose or unavail-

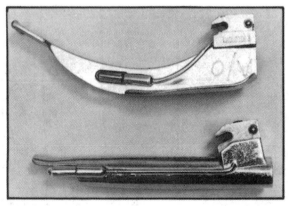

Figure 2-19   Types of laryngoscope blades.

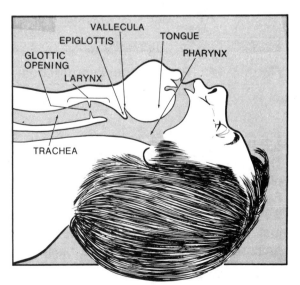

Figure 2-20   Side view of larynx.

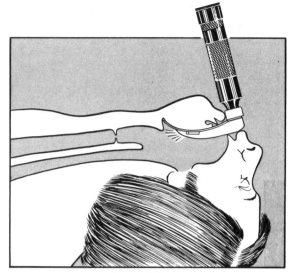

Figure 2-21   Curved laryngoscope blade.

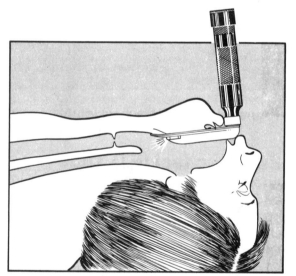

Figure 2-22   Straight laryngoscope blade.

able, the straight blade would be preferred. A common problem during emergency intubation is having the laryngoscope blade light be out due to low batteries. If the light is checked at the beginning of each day or shift, this problem becomes uncommon. Changing the light bulb during a resuscitation attempt is very difficult. It is best to have two laryngoscope blades available— one curved and one straight. One pediatric blade is also useful, but in its absence, a straight adult blade can be used. The goal is to see the cords or at least the arytenoid

cartilage (Figure 2.23). The larynogoscope blade is made to engage the handle at one angle and then to be stable when opened 90 degrees (see Figures 2.24 and 2.25). This step must be practiced repeatedly.

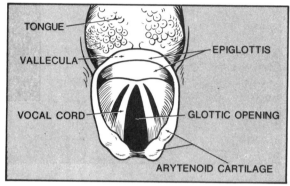

Figure 2-23   Anatomy of glottic opening.

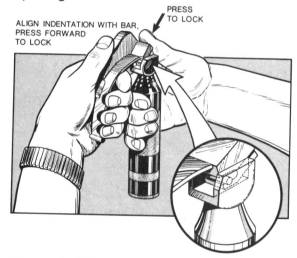

Figure 2-24   Engaging the blade.

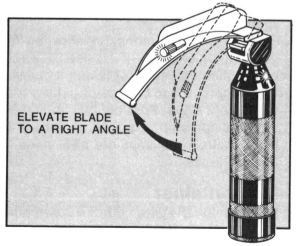

Figure 2-25   Elevating the blade.

Magill Forceps

Magill forceps are rarely needed during oral intubation to place the tip of the tube into the larynx. Since the forceps have teeth, there is a risk of tearing the balloon of the tube.

Occasionally, the Magill forceps may be used to remove foreign bodies lodged in the larynx—but only if they are causing severe distress. In many paramedic programs the Magill forceps is used only to remove foreign material stuck in the airway, not to assist with difficult intubation.

Stylet

In most cases, it is difficult to maneuver the soft tube into the larynx. A stylet can be used to accomplish this placement (Figure 2.26). Because the stylet is firm, it must not be allowed to protrude beyond the tip of the tube. A safer location is about ½ inch back from the tip of the ET tube. To save making this a step in intubation, the stylet should be present for the No. 8 endotracheal tube so that it will not protrude if used. Many manufacturers now have stylets prepackaged inside the tube.

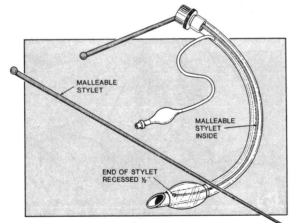

MALLEABLE STYLET

MALLEABLE STYLET INSIDE

END OF STYLET RECESSED ½"

Figure 2–26   The stylet.

Benzoin

Benzoin is a skin adhesive that permits good taping of a tube. It is used in a special applicator to avoid getting it in a patient's eye. A variety of head-encircling clamps are also made to hold ET tubes.

Kit Container

Most items in the paramedic kit are smaller than an intubation kit. The items have to be packaged either in a rolled-up pocket kit or in a flat kit where everything can be seen from above; the latter probably is best.

SKILL SEQUENCE

Check the Equipment

Equipment should be checked at the beginning of every shift (Figures 2.27 to 2.29). First the paramedic must make sure that every item is present. Next, the laryngoscope light must be checked on both blades.

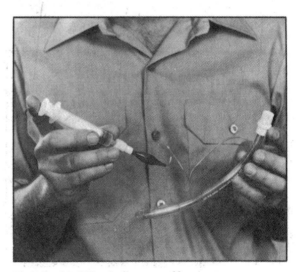

Figure 2–27   Inflate cuff to test.

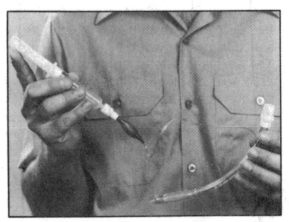

Figure 2–28   Deflate the cuff.

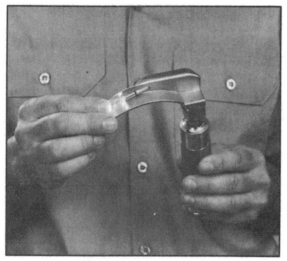

Figure 2–29 Check blade light.

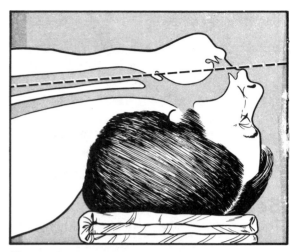

Figure 2–31 Correct "sniff" position.

The balloon is filled with 10 cc of air and then deflated if the tube is accessible through an open—therefore clean but not sterile—package. This step is often done during the procedure because the tubes are prepackaged and sealed to stay clean.

Position the Head

The patient's head is generally elevated with a small pillow or folded towel to achieve the "sniff" position (Figures 2.30 and 2.31). This allows for the most direct view of the larynx. It reminds the paramedic not to try to drop a patient's head over the side of a bed in an emergency situation to improve

visualization since, in fact, visualization is made worse. Even CPR boards with a head depression make the skill harder than does a flat surface.

In case of unconsciousness due to trauma, one must assume a possible cervical spine fracture. Intubation should be attempted with the head in a neutral position. This is accomplished by having an assistant maintain gentle neck traction as the intubation is done.

Monitor the Breathing

A common indication for intubation is a sedative overdose patient who gets pro-

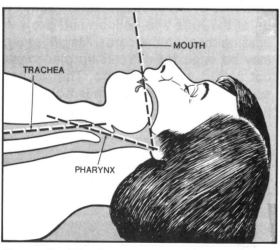

Figure 2–30 Incorrect position.

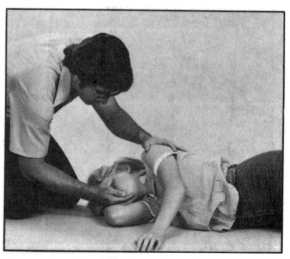

Figure 2–32 Monitor breathing in coma position.

gressively underventilated despite an open airway in the left lateral position. This will best be appreciated by feeling the volume of air exchange on the palm of the hand cupped near the patient's mouth (Figure 2.32).

Test the Lash Reflex

Instead of testing a gag reflex of a patient face up and producing a lethal aspiration, the lash reflex is tried first to estimate activity of reflexes (Figure 2.33). Generally, the lash reflex is sedated at about the same time the gag reflex disappears. (The cough reflex is often still present but does not prevent intubation.) When stroking the eyelids the patient should *not "blink."*

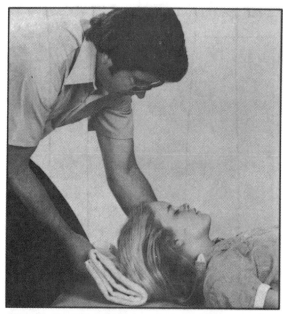

Figure 2–34   Elevate head with towel.

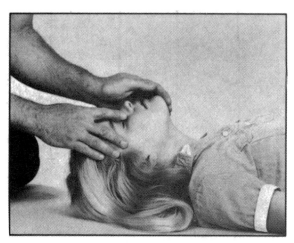

Figure 2–33   Check responsiveness with lash reflex.

hand with a pencil grip to encourage gentle handling. The laryngoscope blade is inserted into the right side of the mouth and then swung to center (Figure 2.35).

Pressure on the teeth is avoided at all times by lifting in the direction the handle is pointing. In a trauma case, the head should be stabilized (Figure 2.36).

Elevate the Head

The head is next elevated with a towel as explained previously (Figure 2.34). Hyperventilate the patient.

Insert the Laryngoscope

The laryngoscope is grasped with the left hand because the flange of the blade is made to push the tongue to the left. The endotracheal tube is grasped with the right

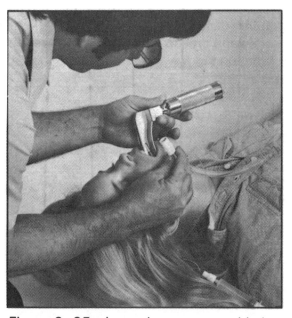

Figure 2–35   Insert laryngoscope blade.

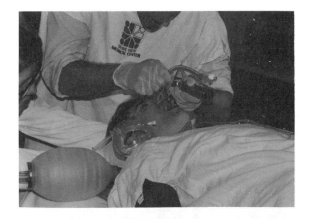

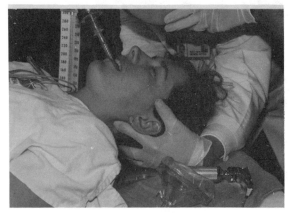

Figure 2–36   Head stabilization in a trauma case.

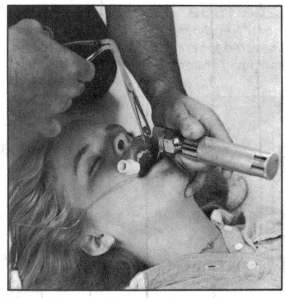

Figure 2–38   Introduce Magill forceps.

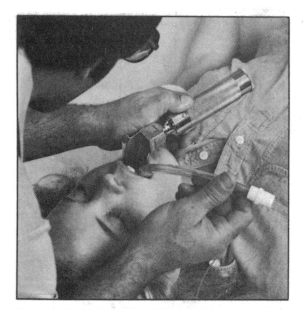

Figure 2–37   Insert ET tube.

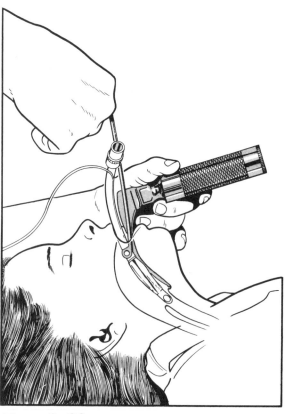

Figure 2–39

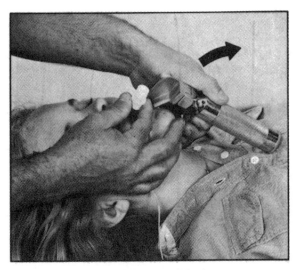

Figure 2–40   Withdraw blade.

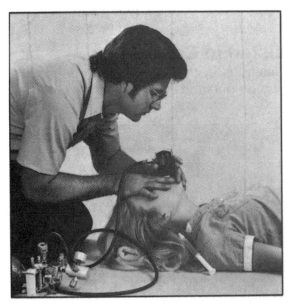

Figure 2–41   Test placement with inflation.

Insert the Tube

When the vocal cords are clearly visualized,
the endotracheal tube should be advanced
starting from the side of the mouth to avoid
obstructing the view (Figure 2.37). The tip
of the tube and balloon cuff are seen passing through the cords. The balloon should
end up only about 1″ past the cords. Magill
forceps may be used for difficult tip
placements not solved with the stylet (Figure
2.38). Avoid placement of the forceps on
the balloon, as perforation may occur. The
laryngoscope is then removed while holding
the tube in place (Figures 2.39 and 2.40).

Seal the Face and Test the Placement

The tube should be tested quickly be sealing the face with cupped hands and blow-
ing into the tube, if alone, or have an assistant ventilate with a positive-pressure
device—bag–valve device for any age or
triggered device for adults (Figure 2.41). If
the chest does not rise, the tube should be
removed and CPR continued until ready for
another attempt. Using this maneuver the

location of the tube can be determined
before inflating the balloon, thus reducing
the time away from CPR.

Resume CPR

CPR should be resumed immediately. The
total time should not exceed 30 seconds. If
the rescuer attemping intubation holds his
or her breath* during the procedure, he or
she is able to estimate the period of time of
patient apnea and will not become oblivious
to time. Make sure that the excited rescuer
does not pass out!

Inflate the Balloon

The balloon should then be inflated and the
syringe removed to allow the one-way valve
to maintain the seal (Figure 2.42). The
balloon should be inflated with 2 to 10 ml
to achieve an air seal. The syring is then
removed.

---

*Exhales and then stops breathing!

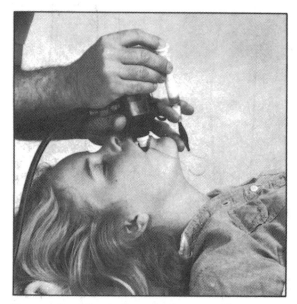

Figure 2-42   Inflate balloon cuff.

Listen to the Chest

Listen to the chest for equal air entry, confirming that the tube is not too far down (Figure 2.43).

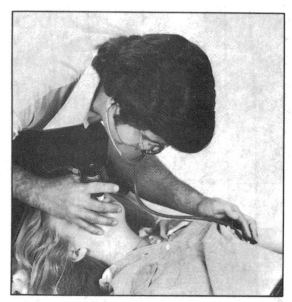

Figure 2-43   Auscultate chest.

Add and Secure the Oropharyngeal Airway

An oropharyngeal airway (OPA) may be used as a bite block to avoid having the patient bite on the tube (Figure 2.44).

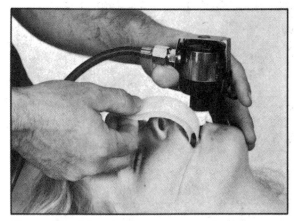

Figure 2-44   Add oropharyngeal airway.

Tape the Tube

The OPA is secured first. Then the ET tube is secured separately with tape or similar device (Figure 2.45). (The use of benzoin is optional.)

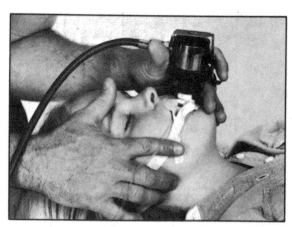

Figure 2-45   Tape tube and OPA separately.

Remove the Tube

In general, an endotracheal tube can be removed when a patient is responsive enough to reach purposefully for the tube. This means that the patient is probably alert enough to cough and move air well. This rule of thumb is commonly used in the postoperative patient in deciding when to extubate (remove the tube). The underlying assumption is that the patient has normal ventilation and can now take over. If the disease process involves damaged lungs, the decision of when it is safe to extubate a patient is more complicated and takes more experience. The rescuer has to make sure the patient will:

1. Be able to keep the airway open

2. Be able to clear secretions with coughing

3. Be able to tolerate 40% oxygen or less

4. Be able to breathe without continuous positive pressure

Although it is possible to deliver high-concentration oxygen and positive pressure through a demand valve and mask, this is not a long-term solution and the patient will be reintubated in the hospital.

The first step in removing the endotracheal tube is to untape the tube and the oral airway. Before the tube is removed preparations are made in case the tube must be replaced. The ET tube cuff is then deflated. The tube is removed during inspiration when the cords are widest (Figure 2.46). Finally, airway maneuvers are used to keep the jaw elevated. Suctioning of the lungs and oropharynx followed by hyperoxygenation prior to removal decreases the likelihood of laryngospasm or hypoxia. Usually, laryngospasm is resolved in about 15 seconds with oxygen.

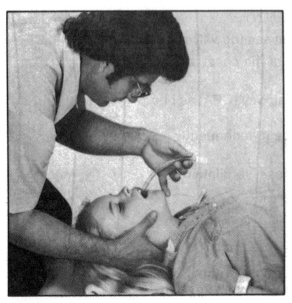

Figure 2-46 Extubate during inspiration.

Infant Endotracheal Intubation

The principal difference between infant and adult endotracheal intubation is that the infant equipment is smaller. Also, since the infant trachea narrows below the vocal cords, the infant ET tube is tapered and no tracheal balloon cuff is needed. Since most infant or child cardiopulmonary arrests begin as respiratory arrests, access to the airway is important.

Most students practice initially on infant intubation manikins. However, sedating kittens with ketamine allows the student to practice intubation where some reflexes are still present. This type of skill experience is very helpful in preparation for the pre-hospital situation.

In urban centers the short transport distances plus the difficulty of doing pediatric skills in the field lead to the common recommendation of using basic skills and transporting pediatric emergencies. Where transport distances are longer, as in a rural setting, advanced skills must be done, but skill maintenance is a bigger problem. Practicing on a monthly basis in a hospital may be the only way to keep up these skills.

Pediatric laryngoscope blades may be kept in the kits, but often the straight adult laryngoscope blade may be used on a child successfully. The size of the endotracheal tube may be estimated from the diameter of the child's index finger. Thus a rapid comparison may be made easily. Table 2.1 (presented earlier in the chapter) provided data on ET tube size and age.

LAB PRACTICE

The following Endotracheal Intubation Procedure Guide and Endotracheal Tube Suctioning Procedure Guide are to be used during lab practice of this skill. Paired students take turns being rescuer and evaluator. The sequences have been set up this time for the CPR situation.

ENDOTRACHEAL INTUBATION PROCEDURE GUIDE

Rescuer's Name _____ Date _____ Evaluator _____

Directions for Evaluator: Place a check beside each item whenever an exam step is omitted, performed improperly, or presented improperly.

Step	Method	Evaluation Adult	Evaluation Infant
1. Check the equipment	a. Check to see if intubation kit is complete.	_____	_____
	b. Test laryngoscope blade light on each blade at beginning of shift.	_____	_____
	c. Remove tube from package, test cuff balloon, and then deflate just prior to use. Keep in clean field.	_____	_____
2. Use the proper grip	a. Engage laryngoscope blade and bring to right angle.	_____	_____
	b. Grasp laryngoscope with left hand and endotracheal tube with right hand.	_____	_____
3. Interrupt CPR	a. Hyperventilate, then tell the rescue crew to stop CPR.	_____	_____
4. Insert the tube	a. Sweep tongue to the left of the patient's mouth with blade.	_____	_____
	b. Visualize vocal cords without undue pressure on teeth.	_____	_____
	c. Insert ET tube until cuff passes cords and remove laryngoscope.	_____	_____
5. Seal the face and test	a. Seal face with hands around tube.	_____	_____
	b. Ventilate and watch chest rise.	_____	_____
6. Resume CPR	a. Resume CPR.	_____	_____
	b. Time limit for stopping CPR less than 30 seconds.	_____	_____

ENDOTRACHEAL INTUBATION PROCEDURE GUIDE
Continued

Step	Method	Evaluation Adult	Infant
7. Inflate the balloon	a. Inflate balloon 5 to 10 ml.*	_____	_____
	b. Remove syringe from sealing valve.*	_____	_____
8. Listen to the chest	a. Listen to both sides of the chest for equal air entry.	_____	_____
9. Add OPA and secure	a. Add oropharyngeal airway (OPA) as bite block.	_____	_____
	b. Secure OPA and tube independently with tape.	_____	_____
10. Ventilate	a. Using a bag–valve–mask, ventilate once every 5 seconds.	_____	_____
11. Remove	a. Untape ET tube and OPA.	_____	_____
	b. Remove OPA.	_____	_____
	c. Suction orophaynx.	_____	_____
	d. Deflate ET tube cuff.*	_____	_____
	e. If patient wakes up, remove tube during inspiration when cords are open.	_____	_____
	f. Keep airway open with jaw maneuvers.	_____	_____

*Not necessary with infant endotrachael intubation.

ENDOTRACHEAL TUBE
SUCTIONING PROCEDURE GUIDE

Rescuer's Name _____ Date _____ Evaluator _____

Directions for Evaluator: Place a check beside each item whenever an exam step is omitted, performed improperly, or presented improperly.

Step	Evaluation
1. Connect suction source.	_____
2. Put on sterile glove (rarely time for this in CPR).	_____
3. Stop CPR.	_____
4. Hyperventilate patient.	_____
5. Grasp suction catheter.	_____
6. Open ventilation system.	_____
7. Advance suction catheter down tube.	_____
8. Close side vent and remove slowly.	_____
9. Close ventilation system.	_____
10. Start CPR.	_____
11. CPR stopped not more than 15 seconds.	_____
12. Side vent not closed more than 5 seconds.	_____

Endotracheal Suctioning

The endotracheal tube offers, over the esophageal obturator airway, the advantage of direct tracheal suctioning. This skill, while important to clear the airway, must be done rapidly since the act of suctioning deprives a patient of air. The very patient who needs suctioning the most is often least able to tolerate it. Experienced critical care professionals know that improper suctioning is a common percursor to cardiac arrest.

JUDGMENT

Indications

Endotrachael suctioning is indicated in a patient if noisy respirations follow the insertion of an endotracheal tube.

Contraindications

If suctioning is done quickly without much pause in ventilation, it is hard to conceive of a valid contraindication. Some teach students to avoid suctioning patients with head injuries regardless of need since this might cause coughing and thus worsen intracranial pressure, but this incorrectly places the priority of central nervous system above that of airway.

Precautions

Make sure that suctioning occurs only as the suction catheter is withdrawn. The procedure should be done with either clean or sterile technique as the situation allows. *Hyperoxgenate before and after suctioning!*

Complications

The complications of endotracheal suctioning are: hypoxia due to prolonged interruption of ventilation, and trauma to trachea if suction pressure is too strong.

EQUIPMENT

Most suction catheters now are equipped with a side vent that allows the operator to control the timing of suctioning (Figure 2.47). A sterile glove is included in the package for use when there is time. The catheter should be no wider than one-third the lumen of the ET tube; generally, a 14 to 16 French size is appropriate for the adult. There are many types of suction sources available.

SKILL SEQUENCE

The following skill sequence integrates the use of suctioning during CPR. The patient is presumed to have been intubated and is being ventilated with high-flow oxygen.

1. Rescuer connects catheter to suction source and turns on suction.

2. Rescuer puts on sterile glove (Figure 2.48).

3. Rescuer grasps suction catheter with sterile glove, doubling it over to prevent the tip from getting contaminated (Figure 2.49).

4. Rescuer stops CPR, separates ventilation device from ET tube, and advances suction catheter down tube until it stops or until it is 5 inches past end of ET tube (Figure 2.50).

5. Rescuer closes side vent and removes catheter slowly, over 5 seconds, using a rotating motion (Figure 2.51).

6. Rescuer resecures ventilation device on ET tube.

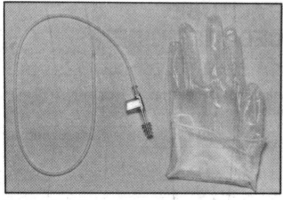

Figure 2-47   Suction catheter kit.

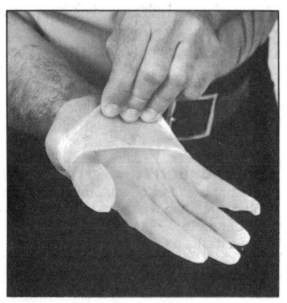

Figure 2-48   Put on sterile glove.

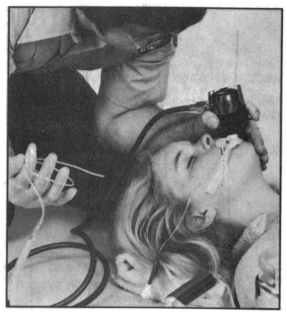

Figure 2–49   Grasp catheter.

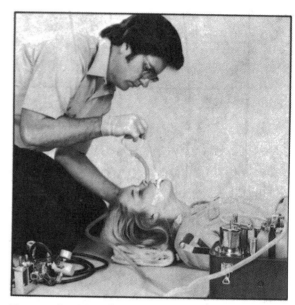

Figure 2–51   Cover vent and remove.

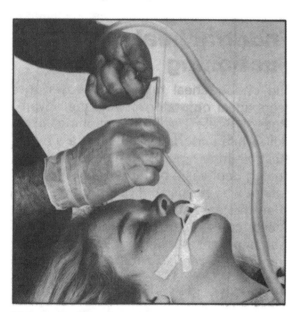

Figure 2–50   Insert catheter.

7. Procedure takes 20 seconds, but CPR is not stopped more than 15 seconds and suctioning is not active for more than 5 seconds.

Nasotracheal Intubation

So far the oral-tracheal form of endotracheal tube intubation has been discussed. Another option for potential field use is nasotracheal intubation (Figures 2.52 and 2.53). In this case a non-precut endotracheal tube, well lubricated with a water-base gel, is advanced from the nose into the trachea.

This advancement almost always involves use of the McGill forceps to enter the trachea correctly. During this step, shown in Figure 2.54, the cuff of the endotracheal tube may be torn and the whole procedure

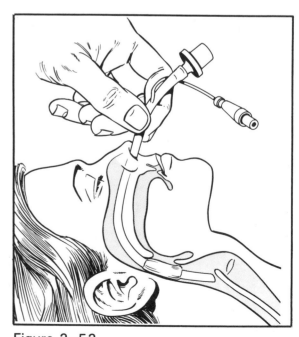

Figure 2–52

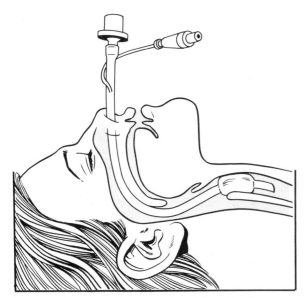

Figure 2–53 Nasotracheal intubation overview.

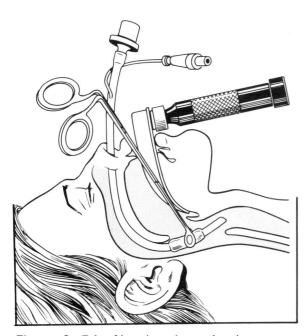

Figure 2–54 Nasal endotracheal.

rendered useless until a new tube can be obtained.

Although the end result is an endotracheal tube that is well secured in the nose and better tolerated by the responsive patient due to less gagging, the potential

problems render the skill difficult for pre-hospital use. These include: nasal hemorrhage, rupture of the cuff balloon, and laryngeal damage due to increased manipulation. However, programs set up with extensive time for training in this area may choose to include this skill.

With proper training a paramedic can become skilled at nasotracheal intubation without visualization, called "blind nasotracheal intubation." The tube is advanced gradually until either the trachea is entered or breath sounds increase in intensity through the tube. If breath sounds heard through the tube suddenly stop even though the patient is still exchanging air, the tube is probably in the esophagus and needs to be repositioned. This approach is useful in trauma since the head may be kept in a neutral position. Its use in head trauma, though, adds the risk of passing the tube through the nose and into the brain through an open basilar skull fracture.

When this skill is attempted on an awake patient, a topical anesthesia such as Cetacaine Spray should be applied to the nose. Neosynephrine spray should be used as well to reduce the size of the nasal mucosa and thus reduce the chance of nasal hemorrhage.

Digital Intubation

An alternative to using the laryngoscope to visualize the opening between the vocal cords—called the *glottis*—is the technique of digital intubation. In this skill, the rescuer feels the epiglottis and guides the tube into the larynx. The rescuer is at the side of the patient. Using the index and long finger of the right hand, the rescuer palpates the epiglottis (Figure 2.55). The tube is then advanced by the rescuer's left hand.

An alternative approach involves primary use of the left hand.* The following steps are recommended in this approach (see Figures 2.56 and 2.57):

*Ron Stewart, "Tactile Orotracheal Intubation," *Annals of Emergency Medicine*, Vol. 13, March 3, 1984.

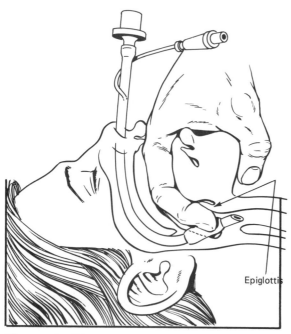

Figure 2–55   Digital intubation using the right hand.

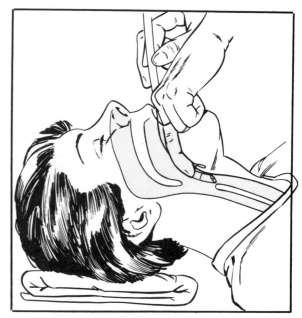

Figure 2–57

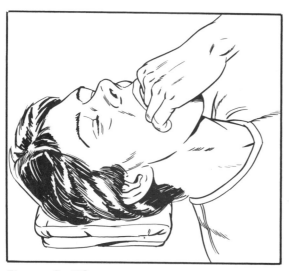

Figure 2–56

1. The endotracheal tube is selected and a stylette is introduced up to the side hole of the tube.

2. The tube is then bent into a "J," particularly so that a gentle hook is produced.

3. The tube is lubricated with a water-base gel.

4. The paramedic, preferably with gloves on, kneels facing the patient with the tube in the right hand.

5. The patient is preoxygenated.

6. The paramedic places the left index and middle fingers of the left hand into the patient's mouth on the patient's right side.

7. The patient's tongue is depressed as the intubator's fingers find the patient's epiglottis in the midline.

8. The tube is then slid along the left side of the patient's mouth and guided toward the epiglottis.

9. The epiglottis is then hooked forward to depress the epiglottis anteriorly.

10. The tube is then directed into the glottis and the stylette removed.

11. The tube is advanced so that the balloon will lie just below the cords.

12. The tube is tested for placement by auscultation and then if correctly placed is secured.

It is most important that the patient be auscultated immediately with ventilation to verify that the tube is truly in the trachea and not in the esophagus. If the tube is in the esophagus, it should be removed and reinserted.

A variety of tubes have been created so that they may be used even with incorrect placement. Their utilization in prehospital care is still being studied.

Securing the Endotracheal Tube

After oral tracheal intubation, the position of the tube with respect to the mouth should be maintained. Usually, this position corresponds to the junction of the small balloon inflation catheter with the larger endotracheal tube lying at the level of the patient's lips. During positive pressure ventilation, this position can easily change unless the tube is secured.

Simple adhesive tape is one option. A half inch or even a full inch of adhesive tape may be used. If the tape is brought all the way around the patient's head, the section of the tape touching the patient's hair should be covered with a shorter piece of tape so that it won't stick to the hair.

An alternative is the use of a predesigned tube stabilization system. One such device is called Endo-Lok. The equipment is pictured in Figure 2.58. Application involves the following four steps:

1. Slip the open side of the bite block around the endotracheal tube without jostling the tube (Figure 2.59).

2. Apply the foam pad fabric side down between the patient's chin and the support bar and then loop the small strap around the tube (Figure 2.60);

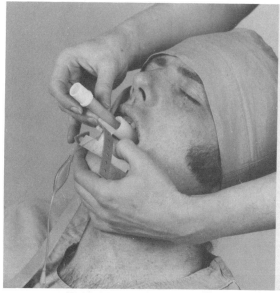

Figure 2–59   Securing the endotracheal tube.

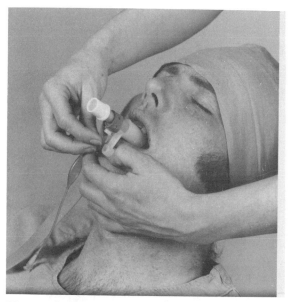

Figure 2–60   Securing the endotracheal tube.

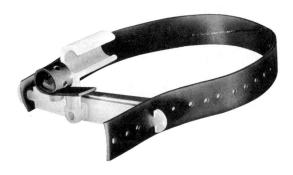

Figure 2–58   Endo-Lok.

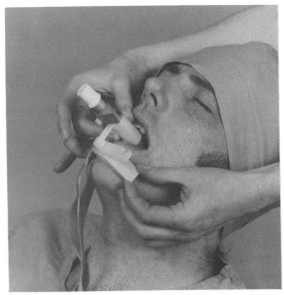

Figure 2-61 Securing the endotracheal tube.

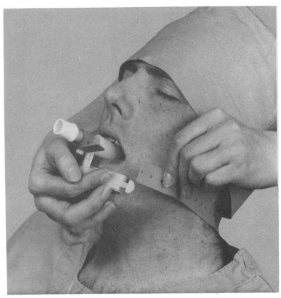

Figure 2-62 Securing the endotracheal tube.

3. Place the headstrap below the patient's mouth and under the patient's ears, and behind the patient's head (Figure 2.61); or

4. Place the strap over the patient's upper lip and around above the patient's ears (Figure 2.62).

This should only be done after the position of the ET tube has been determined to be correct.

When time is critical, the paramedic ventilating the patient may simply choose to hold the tube and cup the patient's chin. This is usually done with the left hand so that ventilation can occur with the right.

Percutaneous Cricothyrotomy

The larynx lies just below the skin at the level of the cricothyroid membrane (Figure 2.63). This is the small depression that may be felt just below the thyroid cartilage (Adam's apple). This area is relatively free of blood vessels and offers a site for entrance to the airway just below the vocal cords.

A number of approaches may be used to create a cricothyroid airway. The first is the use of a simple straight IV catheter-needle, where the catheter is left in place and the needle withdrawn. The second involves a specially designed curved needle prepared for cricothyrotomy (shown in Chapter 3 under the subject of percutaneous transtracheal ventilation [PTV]).

The third approach involves using one of several specially prepared cricothyroid kits, which allow placement of fairly large airways. One example, the Nu-Trake, is

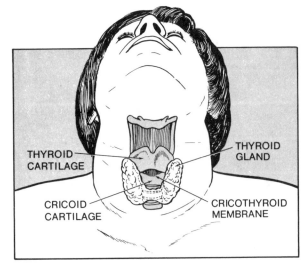

Figure 2-63 Anatomy of the cricothyroid membrane.

shown in this chapter. Finally, the surgical approach allows placement of the full tracheostomy-type tube and is also shown.

Whatever is used, once completely obstructed, the airway must be entered within a matter of minutes. Equipment should be preselected and stored for easy retrieval.

JUDGMENT

Indications

Cricothyrotomy is used only for complete airway obstruction with progressive cyanosis or with cardiopulmonary arrest. It is an extraordinary skill requiring special training and skill maintenance. It is tried only after other approaches, such as endotracheal intubation, have failed.

Contraindications

As this is a life-or-death skill, it is hard to place specific contraindications. Certainly lack of training, however, would be one. The procedure is especially difficult if the patient has a large, thick neck or has a tendency to bleed.

Precautions

The rescuer must not push too deep when entering the cricothyroid membrane since injury to the softer posterior wall can occur and lead to a false passage. The tube should not be assumed to be in correct position until air exchange is achieved spontaneously or artificially with positive pressure.

Complications

Potential complications include creation of a false passage with development of subcutaneous emphysema and mediastinal emphysema, damage to the vocal cords and larynx, and introduction of bleeding into an already compromised airway.

EQUIPMENT

A visual overview of cricothyrotomy with the Nu-Trach device is shown in Figures 2.64 to 2.66. As will be shown, the sharp stylette is replaced in several steps with an airway tube.

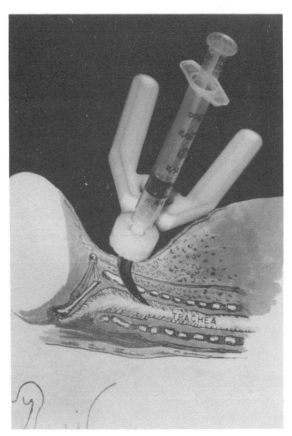

Figure 2–64

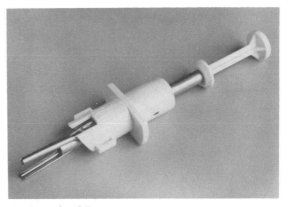

Figure 2–65

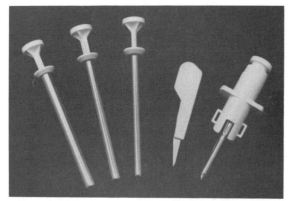

Figure 2-66

Nu-Trach for adults and Pedia-Trake for children each come as prepackaged, sterile kits. The adult Nu-Trach is pictured in Figure 2.67. Several sizes of obturators—2.8 mm, 4.5 mm, and 8 mm—are available. The Pedia-Trake comes with a special set of handles to allow spreading of the needle halves (Figure 2.68).

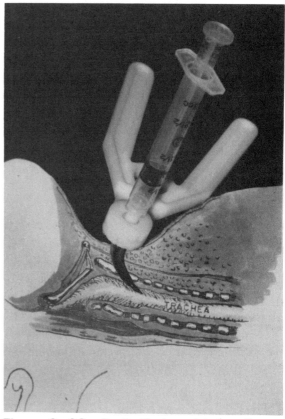

Figure 2-68   Pedia-Trake with handles.

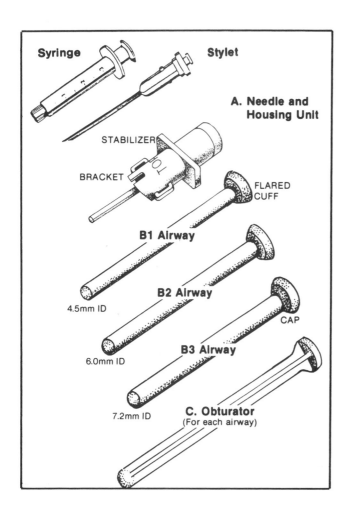

Figure 2-67   Nu-Trake. (A) The stylet has an accurate point to facilitate its passage through the tissues. The needle is divided lengthwise and held together by an elastic "O" band to accommodate airways of various sizes. The tubular housing unit is designed to rest on the cricoid cartilage; the lower edge is slanted to approximate the entrance angle of the needle. Stabilizers steady the instrument for one-hand operation, while brackets on the sides hold the ties used to secure the instrument. Airway and obturator are inserted through the opening at the distal end of the housing.   (B) The flared cuff prevents over descent into the housing and aids in removal. The particular size airway to be used is dependent upon estimated trachea size.   (C) The obturator acts as a plunger to facilitate introduction of the airway and prevent clogging with tissue particles. The cap is designed for easy removal.

Both the Pedia-Trach and the Nu-Trach come with a universal adapter allowing positive-pressure ventilation to occur either by mouth-to-mouth technique or by the use of other devices. If the patient still has a respiratory drive, positive pressure may not be needed.

SKILL SEQUENCE— NU-TRACH (ADULT)

Check the Equipment

Since the Nu-Trach comes prepackaged, the equipment is essentially together. If there is time—and usually there is not—the neck could be swabbed with alcohol or iodine.

Procedure*

STEP ONE. Patient's neck is hyperextended, if possible, and cricothyroid membrane identified. The knife blade should incise the skin 1 to 2 cm (Figure 2.69).

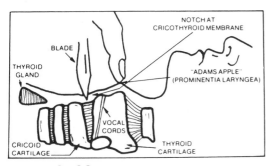

Figure 2–69

STEP TWO. The needle should puncture the membrane just beyond entry at approximately the same angle as the lower edge of the housing (Figure 2.70). Expulsion of air indicates tracheal entrance.

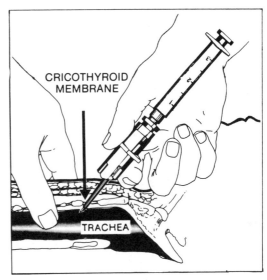

Figure 2–70

STEP THREE. The stylet is removed. The blunt needle is gently moved farther into the trachea until the housing rests on the overlying skin (Figure 2.71).

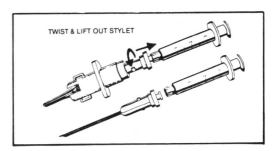

Figure 2–71

*Specific skill steps used with slight adaptations from the manufacturer's literature, with permission.

STEP FOUR. A freely rocking motion confirms proper depth of insertion (Figure 2.72).

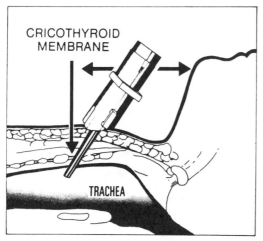

Figure 2–72

STEP FIVE. Airway and obturator are inserted together into the distal end of the housing unit. Use the B1 airway (OD 4 mm) first in all cases. Index and middle fingers grasp the housing below the stabilizers, with the thenar eminence resting against the cap of the obturator (Figure 2.73). Airway and obturator together are *pushed* (not squeezed) downward into the needle, which is divided lengthwise and spreads apart to accommodate them.

STEP SIX. Obturator is removed, leaving a clear passage for air to reach the lungs. If airway size requires change, this can be easily performed by leaving the housing and needle guide in place, while insertion of various airways are made. Ties are threaded through brackets on sides of housing (Figure 2.74).

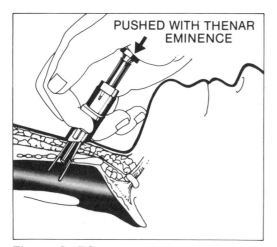

Figure 2–73

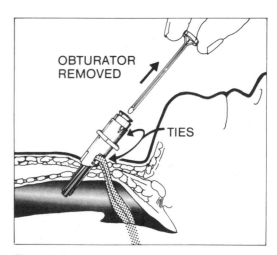

Figure 2–74

SYSTEM IN OPERATION. Universal adapter may be fitted to the top of housing (Figure 2.75). Expansion of lungs can be started by mouth-to-airway respiration, with fingers closing off the vents in the housing.

STEP TWO. Hold trachea with hand. Puncture membrane with needle. Easy-moving syringe obturator denotes tracheal entrance (Figure 2.77).

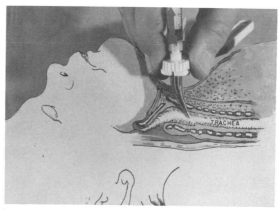

Figure 2–77

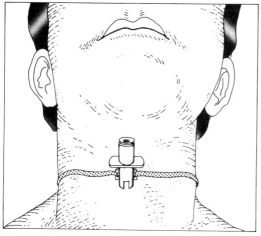

Figure 2–75

SKILL SEQUENCE—
Pedia Trake

STEP THREE. Rotate locking collar and disengage the stylet and syringe (Figure 2.78).

STEP ONE. Hyperextend head if possible. Incise skin overlying cricothyroid membrane 1 to 2 cm (Figure 2.76).

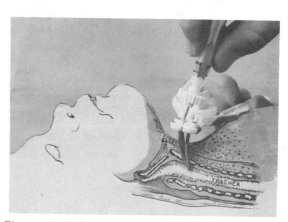

Figure 2–78

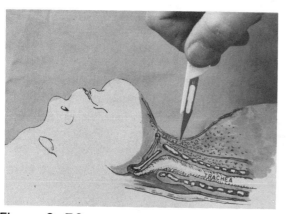

Figure 2–76

STEP FOUR. Move blunt needle further, gently. Rotate needle tip slightly upward. Squeeze handles to accommodate proper tube size (Figure 2.79).

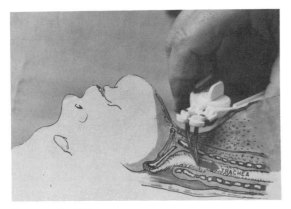

Figure 2-79

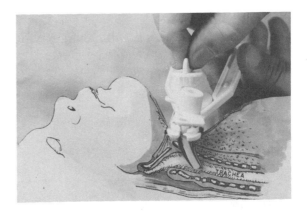

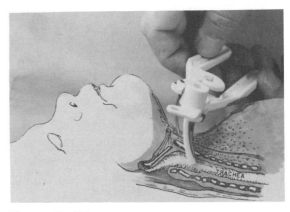

Figure 2-81

STEP FIVE. Insert tracheal tube. Remove obturator. Maintain instrument in place until medically sound to remove. Secure instrument and tube with ties (Figure 2.80).

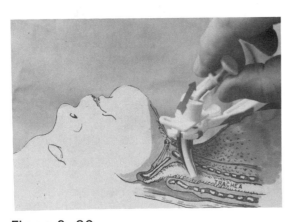

Figure 2-80

STEP SIX. Removal of Instrument. Turn locking key counterclockwise and remove. Remove handle 1. Remove handle 2 (Figure 2.81).

Surgical Cricothyrotomy

Surgical cricothyrotomy requires more equipment, steps, and therefore skill. The principal advantage over the percutaneous approach is the direct visualization of the airway opening and the opportunity to place a larger tube into the airway. Familiarity with the equipment might help the paramedic deal with a partially lacerated anterior neck with airway compromise.

The indications, contraindications, and precautions are the same as with percutaneous cricothyrotomy. The anatomy needs to be understood more thoroughly and is portrayed in Figure 2.82.

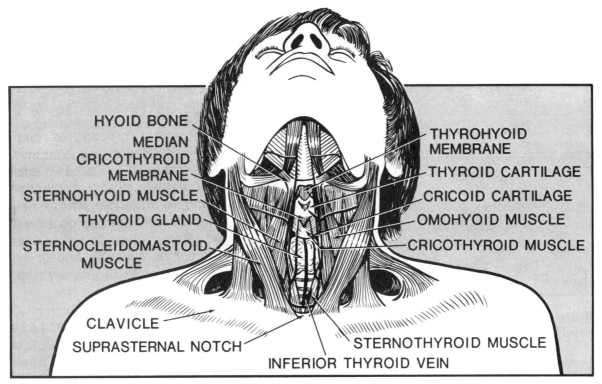

Figure 2–82   Front view of larynx.

Complications

The possible complications of surgical cricothyrotomy include false passage, bleeding, damage to the larynx and vocal cords, subcutaneous emphysema, mediastinal emphysema, and so forth.

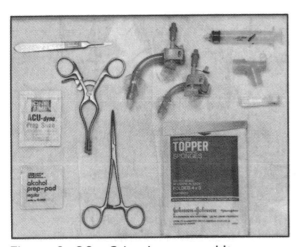

Figure 2–83   Cricothyrotomy kit.

EQUIPMENT

There are many cricothyrotomy kits available. Most involve the following features: scissors to cut the skin, a pointed tool to puncture the membrane, a spreading mechanism to enlarge the hole, and an airway tube for the new passageway. The various kits try to combine these functions for the most efficient use. A kit using common hospital surgical instruments is shown in Figure 2.83.

SKILL SEQUENCE

Examine the Kit (Beginning of Shift)

Examine kit prior to packing it in the rescue box. Make sure that the kit includes:

1.   Iodine swabs for preparing the skin

2. Device for opening the skin and membrane

3. Device for widening orifice (hole)

4. Airway tube—at least a No. 4 size

Try the Basic Maneuvers

Make sure that all manual maneuvers for improving the airway have been used, including direct visualization with a laryngoscope and attempt at airway improvement with a Magill forceps, removing the foreign body if indicated.

Hyperextend the Neck

Hyperextend the neck (unless cervical injury suspected) by placement of a large rolled-up towel behind the neck horizontally or vertically between the shoulder blades (Figure 2.84).

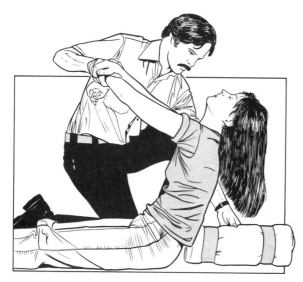

Figure 2–84   Place rolled-up towel under neck and upper back.

Identify the Membrane

Identify the thyroid cartilage (Adam's apple) and the cricoid cartilage with the left hand anteriorly. Now locate the cricothyroid membrane between these two landmarks (Figure 2.85). Hold the trachea with the thumb and

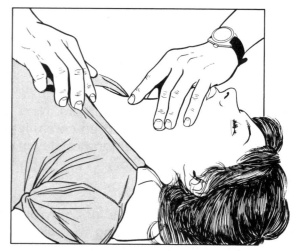

Figure 2–85   Identify cricothyroid anatomy.

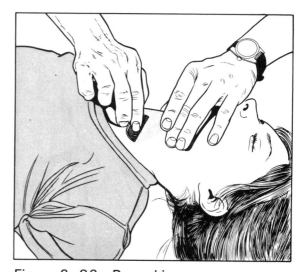

Figure 2–86   Prep skin.

long finger of the left hand, leaving the index finger free to identify the cricothyroid membrane.

Prep the Neck

Prep the neck with iodine if the patient's condition permits (Figure 2.86).

Incise the Skin and the Membrane

Incise the skin transversely 2.5 cm. Next spread the skin with a retractor. Then carefully incise the cricothyroid membrane. Stay in the midline (Figures 2.87 to 2.89).

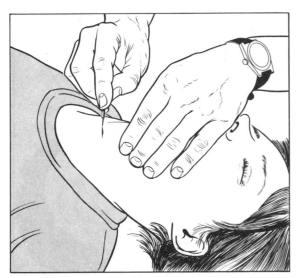

Figure 2–87   Incise skin.

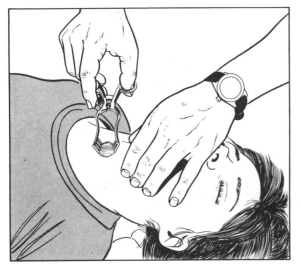

Figure 2–88   Apply skin retractor.

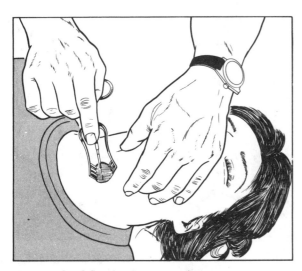

Figure 2–89   Incise membrane.

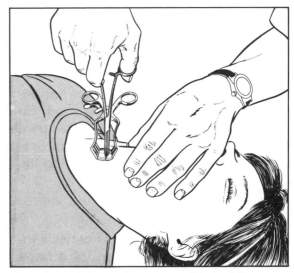

Figure 2–90   Enlarge opening with Mayo clamp.

Enlarge the Hole

Enlarge the orifice of the cricothyroid membrane using a spreading tool such as a Mayo clamp (Figure 2.90).

Insert the Tube

Insert a tracheotomy tube of at least size No. 4, directing it inferiorly. Then remove stylus, inflate balloon, and remove syringe (Figures 2.91 to 2.95).

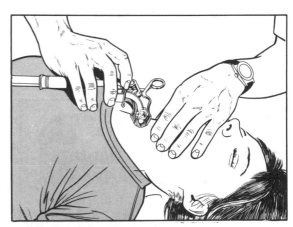

Figure 2–91   Insert tracheotomy tube— early.

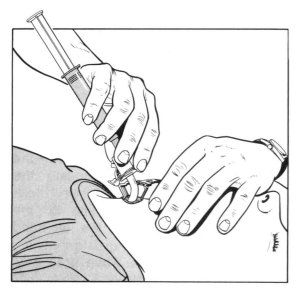

Figure 2–92   Insert tracheotomy tube—mid.

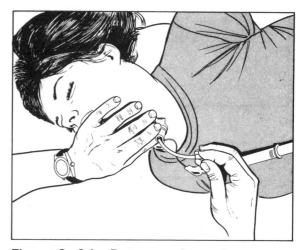

Figure 2–94   Remove tybe stylus.

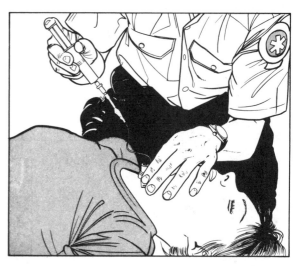

Figure 2–95   Inflate balloon.

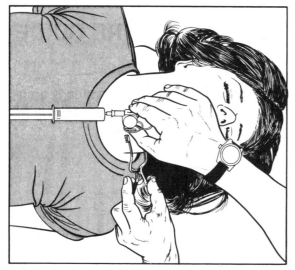

Figure 2–93   Insert tracheotomy tube—late.

Ventilate and Auscultate

Make sure that there is easy airflow through the tube; if unclear, ventilate patient and listen for equal air entry on both sides of the chest (Figure 2.96).

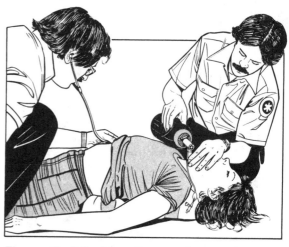

Figure 2–96   Ventilate and auscultate.

Secure the Tube

Secure the airway tube using square knots, since bow ties may slip and light plastic tubes can be expelled during coughing. Do not cut the gauze pad since fibers may enter the trachea. Fold instead (Figures 2.97 to 2.99).

LAB PRACTICE

The following Surgical Cricothyrotomy Procedure Guide is to be used during lab practice of this skill. Paired students take turns being rescuer and evaluator. The sequence has been set up for a patient with facial trauma preventing an adequate airway.

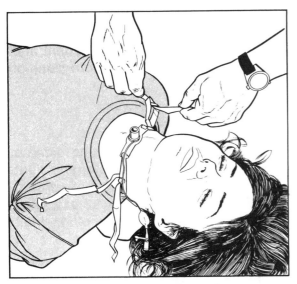

Figure 2-97   Tie with square knots to secure.

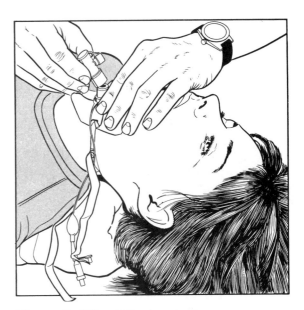

Figure 2-99   Attach adapter.

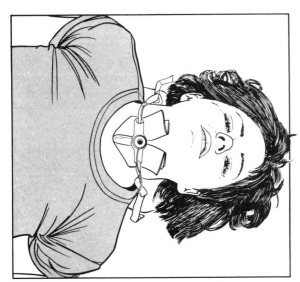

Figure 2-98   Complete with folded gauze pad.

SURGICAL CRICOTHYROTOMY PROCEDURE GUIDE

Rescuer's Name_____ Date_____ Evaluator_____

Directions for Evaluator: Place a check beside each item whenever an exam step is omitted, performed improperly, or presented improperly.

Step	Evaluation
1. Examine kit for completeness.	_____
2. Place roll under back and neck.	_____
3. Identify cricothyroid membrane.	_____
4. Prep skin.	_____
5. Incise skin.	_____
6. Apply skin retractor.	_____
7. Incise membrane.	_____
8. Enlarge opening with Mayo clamp.	_____
9. Insert tracheostomy tube.	_____
10. Remove tube stylus.	_____
11. Inflate cuff balloon.	_____
12. Ventilate and auscultate.	_____
13. Secure with square knots.	_____
14. Place gauze pad.	_____
15. Attach swivel adapter.	_____

PTL Airway

Another airway of interest is the pharyngeo-tracheal lumen (PTL) airway (Figure 2.100). It utilizes the principle that the tube can be used whether or not it ends up in the trachea or esophagus. It is undergoing clinical evaluation.

LAB PRACTICE

The following Detailed Inhalation Analgesia Guide is provided as an aid to lab practice of this skill. The lab is to be done in simulated fashion, *not* actually using nitrous oxide.

SUMMARY

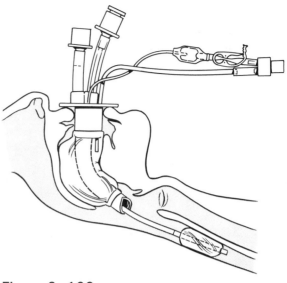

Figure 2–100

Advanced airway skills represent invasive techniques using needles, tubes, or catheters. They are indicated for patients in CPR, patients in deep coma with poor ventilation, or patients with progressive cyanosis from impaired airway. Used in these circumstances, the benefits outweigh the risks. The more rarely these skills are used in the field, the more emphasis must be placed on postgraduate ongoing training and testing.

DETAILED INHALATION ANALGESIA GUIDE

Rescuer's Name_____ Date_____ Evaluator_____

Directions for Evaluator: Place a check beside each item whenever an exam step is omitted, performed improperly, or presented improperly.

Sample Patient Problem: a 24-year-old male with a fractured femur from a motorcycle accident. Patient is not in shock. The base hospital has ordered inhalation analgesia.

Step	Method	Evaluation
1. Confirm the order	a. Rescuer determines if order is consistent with training.	_____
	b. Confirms order.	_____
2. Prepare the medication	a. Rescuer checks tanks and mask.	_____
3. Administer the medication	a. Turns on both tanks.	_____
	b. Explains procedure to patient.	_____
	c. Assists patient.	_____
	d. Does not hold mask for patient.	_____
	e. Reports to base hospital, including new vitals and level of consciousness.	_____
4. Confirm administration		

SKILL PROFICIENCY TESTING

Skill Esophageal Obturator Airway Insertion

Performance Demonstrate how to prepare, insert, secure, and later remove an esophageal obturator airway in an adult intubation manikin.

Conditions
1. Simulated CPR is occurring with an adult intubation manikin.

2. Esophageal obturator airway kit is available.

3. Rescuer comes into the room and is told that he or she has just received an order from the base hospital to insert an esophageal obturator airway after checking the equipment.

Standard
1. Rescuer follows Esophageal Airway Procedure Guide, missing no more than five steps. ☐

2. CPR is not interrupted for more than 15 seconds. ☐

Student's Name_____ Date_____ Evaluator_____

Pass/Fail

SKILL PROFICIENCY TESTING

Skill   Adult Endotracheal Intubation (Figure 2.101)

Performance   Demonstrate how to prepare, insert, test, secure, and later remove a No. 8 oral endotracheal tube in an adult intubation manikin.

Conditions

1. Simulated CPR is occurring on an adult intubation manikin.

2. Complete intubation kit is available (a large blade is required for the Laerdal manikin).

3. Laryngoscope and handle are separated within the kit.

4. Chest plate of the manikin is removed so that lung inflation can be viewed by the rescuer.

5. Rescuer comes into the room and is told that he or she has just received an order from the base hospital to insert an endotracheal tube after checking the equipment.

Standard

1. Rescuer follows Endotracheal intubation Procedure Guide, missing no more than five steps.   ☐

2. CPR is not interrupted for more than 30 seconds.   ☐

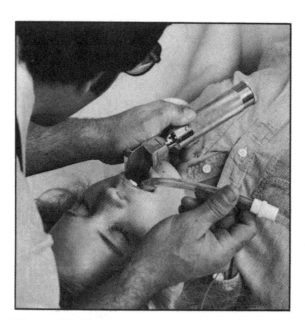

Figure 2–101

Student's Name_____ Date_____ Evaluator_____

SKILL PROFICIENCY TESTING

Skill   Infant Endotracheal Intubation

Performance   Demonstrate how to prepare, insert, test, secure, and later remove a No. 3 endotracheal tube in an infant manikin.

Conditions

1. Simulated CPR is occurring on an infant intubation manikin.

2. Complete pediatric intubation kit is available.

3. The laryngoscope and handle are separated within the kit.

4. Rescuer comes into the room and is told that he or she has just received an order from the base hospital to insert an endotracheal tube after checking the equipment.

Standard

1. Rescuer follows Endotracheal Intubation Procedure Guide, missing no more than five steps.   ☐

2. CPR not interrupted for more than 30 seconds.   ☐

Student's Name_____ Date_____ Evaluator_____

Pass/Fail

SKILL PROFICIENCY TESTING

Skill Endotracheal Suctioning (Figure 2.102)

Performance Demonstrate how to suction mucus properly from a patient with a secured endotracheal tube.

Conditions
1. Intubation manikin on a table with an endotracheal tube already in place.

2. Suction source, suction catheter with "Y" or side vent, and sterile glove all available.

3. Rescuer comes into the room and is told that there is excess mucus in the endotracheal tube and bronchial tree.

Standard
1. Rescuer follows Endotracheal Suctioning Procedure Guide, missing no more than two steps. ☐

2. Rescuer does not interrupt CPR for more than 15 seconds. ☐

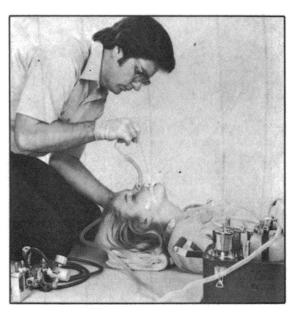

Figure 2–102

Student's Name_____ Date_____ Evaluator_____

Pass/Fail

SKILL PROFICIENCY TESTING

Skill Surgical Cricothyrotomy (Figure 2.103)

Performance Rescuer demonstrates how to perform an emergency cricothyrotomy on an anesthetized dog or suitable manikin.

Conditions 1. Anesthetized dog on operating area is available or a larynx is simulated.

2. Cricothyrotomy kit, including tracheostomy tube, is available.

3. Rescuer comes into the room and is told that he or she has just received an order from the base hospital to perform a surgical cricothyrotomy after checking the equipment.

Standard Rescuer follows Surgical Cricothyrotomy Procedure Guide, missing no more than two steps. ☐

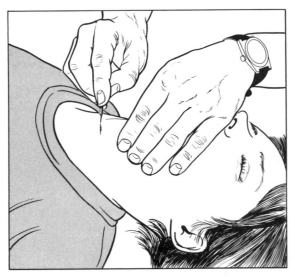

Figure 2–103

Student's Name_____ Date_____ Evaluator_____

Pass/Fail

3

Breathing Skills

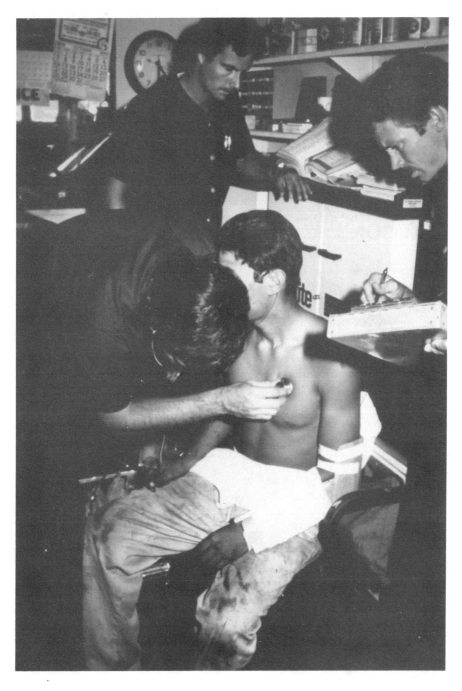

Skills Objectives

- **Pleural Decompression**—Demonstrate how to decompress the pleura in a simulated tension pneumothorax using needle or tube thoracostomy.

- **Percutaneous Transtracheal Ventilation (PVT)**—Demonstrate how to perform a percutaneous transtracheal ventilation.

Outline

Breathing Skills Description

Pleural Decompression
Percutaneous Transtracheal Ventilation

Skill Proficiency Testing

Introduction
Special Considerations

Judgment
Equipment
Skill Sequence
Lab Practice

Breathing Skills Description

INTRODUCTION

Breathing represents the *mechanics* of moving air with sufficient oxygen in and out of the lungs. Breathing cannot occur without the availability of an open airway or passageway into the trachea. Breathing represents the second part of the ABC sequence and is therefore the second priority in patient care.

The basic-level breathing skills covered in the *Basic Life Support Skills Manual* include the following: oxygen by mask, mouth-to-mouth ventilation, demand valve ventilation, and mouth-to-mask ventilation. These skills cover many of the breathing needs of patients and are used routinely by rescuers at all levels.

At the advanced level, breathing skills are of five types:

1. Drugs aimed at reducing fluid backup from the circulation into the alveoli (pulmonary edema)

2. Drugs aimed at reducing bronchospasm

3. Pleural decompression to treat tension pneumothorax

4. Transtracheal oxygen insufflation

In this book drug administration technique is covered in Chapter 5, but specific drugs are not discussed in detail. These should be studied in assessment or theory texts. Therefore, the three advanced breathing skills that will be developed are the application of rotating tourniquets, pleural decompression, and transtracheal oxygen insufflation.

SPECIAL CONSIDERATIONS

Normal Breathing

For normal breathing to occur, the following factors must be present:

1. Impulse from the base of the brain to the muscles of breathing, particularly the diaphragm, to contract

2. Mechanical ability of the diaphragm to flatten, chest wall to expand, and lungs to expand

3. Open airway for air with oxygen under atmospheric pressure to fill the lungs

4. Thin barrier from alveoli to lung capillaries for oxygen and carbon dioxide to pass through in opposite directions

5. Normal lung perfusion with sufficient hemoglobin to pick up the oxygen

6. Normal circulation to get oxygen to the cells

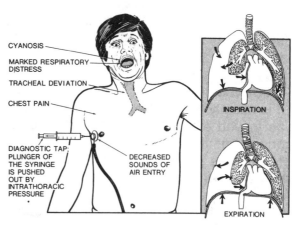

Figure 3–1   Tension pneumothorax.

Conditions

While there are hundreds of breathing conditions, the four common adult conditions in which paramedic intervention can be dramatic include:

1. Asthma, which is generally treated with subcutaneous epinephrine and fluids

2. Emphysema with acute bronchitis, which is generally treated with fluids, low-flow oxygen, and bronchodilators

3. Pulmonary edema, which is generally treated with oxygen, morphine, Lasix, aminophylline, and rarely, rotating tourniquets

4. Tension pneumothorax, which is often relieved with pleural decompression

Pleural Decompression

One of the true lifesaving maneuvers in medicine is the relief of a tension pneumothorax (Figure 3.1). Although this skill has been used by military medics for years with relative safety, its civilian use by paramedics has been approached cautiously.

Tension pneumothorax occurs when air is drawn into a pleural space with each inspiration but does not get back out during expiration. This can occur with a one-way valve system and is caused either by a hole in the chest wall or by an internal air leak from the lung. As pressure increases, cardiorespiratory compromise occurs. The pressure rapidly exceeds the blood pressure and blood return to the chest is compromised. The patient becomes cyanotic, confused, demonstrates signs of shock, and may thrash wildly prior to becoming unconscious.

Although a variety of conditions can lead to a tension pneumothorax, the most common is a penetrating wound of the chest caused by a sharp, icepick-type object or low-velocity bullet, followed by the dramatic clinical picture described above. The physical exam should reveal cyanosis, neck vein distension, tracheal shift, and absent breath sounds on one side of the chest.

At first, the pressure is relieved by releasing the air through a needle or small tube. (Later, in the hospital, a chest tube is inserted.) The paramedic who performs the skill will hear a loud hissing as the air is released, combined with signs of immediate patient relief.

JUDGMENT

Indications

A patient is suspected of having tension pneumothorax when he shows signs of progressive cyanosis (despite a patent airway), shifted trachea, and unequal air entry upon auscultation of the chest.

Contraindications

If the skill is reserved for the clinical picture described above, there are few contraindications other than insufficient training.

Precautions

The chest should be entered in the fourth interspace midaxillary line, even with the supine nipple line (Figure 3.2).

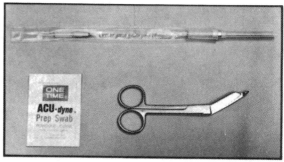

Figure 3–3   Large intercath needle thoracostomy kit.

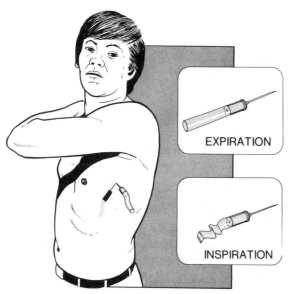

Figure 3–2   Needle thoracostomy.

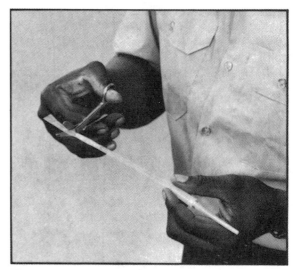

Figure 3–4   Cut intercath plastic sleeve.

Complications

Bleeding from an intercostal artery, lung puncture, and hitting a pulmonary vessel are possible complications.

EQUIPMENT—NEEDLE

One of the easiest devices to use is a normal intercath needle (large size) in which the plastic flashback pocket has been cut and the catheter removed (Figures 3.3 to 3.5).

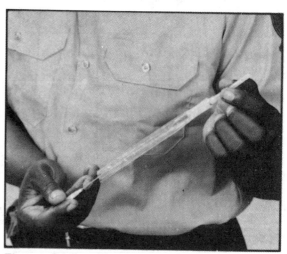

Figure 3–5   Remove stylette.

In this way the paramedic has a needle attached to a simple flutter valve. (A small chest tube nick-named "dart" is currently off of the market due to high insurance costs.)

SKILL SEQUENCE— NEEDLE

The situation would often involve a patient who has had a penetrating wound to the chest which produced gasping respirations, shifted trachea, and unequal air entry (Figure 3.6). The base hospital might elect to order pleural decompression.

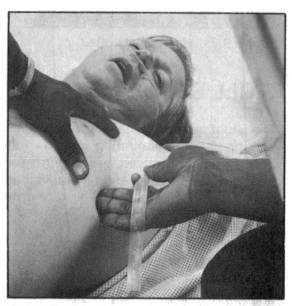

Figure 3–7   Palpate correct interspace.

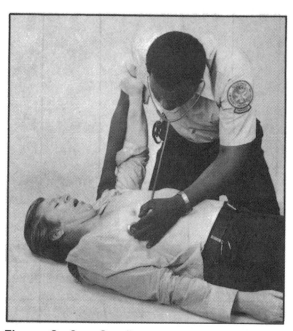

Figure 3–6   Confirm unequal air entry.

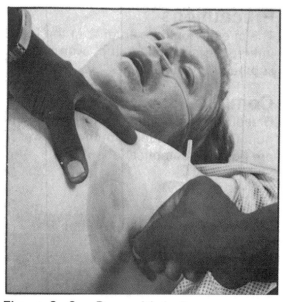

Figure 3–8   Prep with Iodine.

Introduce Self

The paramedic begins with introduction and reassurance.

Palpate and Prep

The paramedic palpates the correct fourth interspace midaxillary line and preps the area with an iodine prep pack (Figures 3.7 and 3.8).

Insert the Needle

The precut large intercath is removed from the paramedic kit and brought to the chest wall. The paramedic asks the patient to hold still as the needle is rapidly pushed through the pleura just over the fifth rib. The undersurface of the fourth rib is avoided so that the neurovascular bundle is not cut (Figs. 3.9 to 3.14).

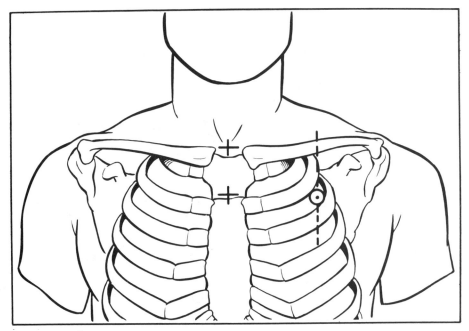

Figure 3-9

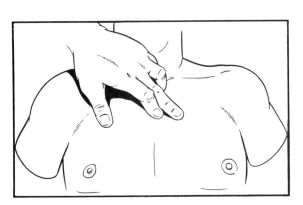

Figure 3-10

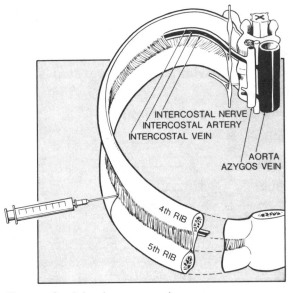

Figure 3-11 Intercostal anatomy.

INTERCOSTAL NERVE
INTERCOSTAL ARTERY
INTERCOSTAL VEIN

AORTA
AZYGOS VEIN

4th RIB

5th RIB

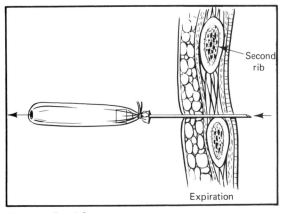

Figure 3-12

Second rib

Expiration

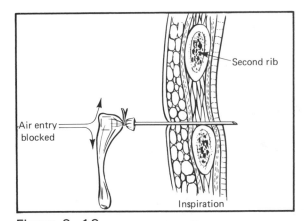

Figure 3-13

Second rib

Air entry blocked

Inspiration

102

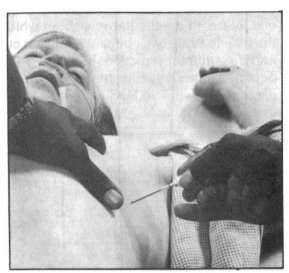

Figure 3–14   Insert needle.

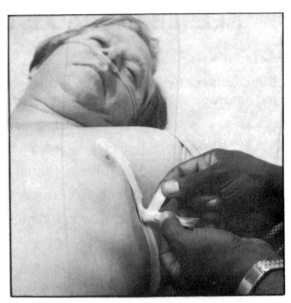

Figure 3–16   Tape flutter valve in place.

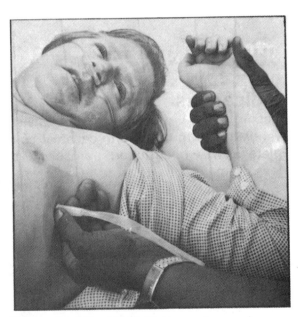

Figure 3–15   Hold flutter valve and check pulse.

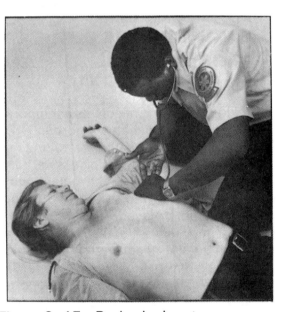

Figure 3–17   Recheck air entry.

Recheck the Patient

The patient should be rechecked for return of equal air entry on auscultation.

LAB PRACTICE—NEEDLE

The following Needle Thoracostomy Procedure Guide is to be used during lab practice of this skill. Students take turns being rescuer, evaluator, and patient.

Check and Tape

Air should escape rapidly. While holding the flutter valve in place, check for improvement in the pulse. Then tape the needle hub in place, avoiding tape on the areola (Figs. 3.15 to 3.17).

NEEDLE THORACOSTOMY PROCEDURE GUIDE

Rescuer's Name _____ Date _____ Evaluator _____

Directions for Evaluator: Place a check beside each item whenever an exam step is omitted, performed improperly, or presented improperly.

Step	**Evaluation**
1. Prepare kit from intercath.	_____
2. Confirm unequal air entry.	_____
3. Palpate correct interspace.	_____
4. Prep with iodine.	_____
5. Insert needle.	_____
6. Check radial pulse.	_____
7. Tape flutter valve in place.	_____
8. Recheck air entry.	_____

Percutaneous Transtracheal Ventilation (PTV)

The idea of using a needle as a temporary airway has been debated vigorously. The debate centers on whether or not the needle, even No. 12, provides a large enough opening for effective ventilation. Many who have tried to breathe through such a needle placed at their lips have found it impossible. Ventilating the patient through such a needle using a high-flow oxygen system has proved effective. The National Academy of Sciences reported that this was an appropriate paramedic skill. Finally, a negative pressure system was added to aid exhalation of carbon dioxide.* The skill is now referred to as PTV (percutaneous transtracheal ventilation), one step of which is needle cricothyrostomy.

*L. B. Dunlop, "A Modified, Simple Device for the Emergency Administration of Percutaneous Transtracheal Ventilation," *JACEP*, Vol. 7, 1978, pp. 42–46.

JUDGMENT

Indications

Needle cricothyrostomy with transtracheal ventilation is to be used in cases of complete airway obstruction unresolved by less dramatic measures. It has been recommended for use in CPR where vomitus or blood fills the pharynx and endotracheal intubation has failed or is not allowed.

Contraindications

If reserved for these near-death situations, contraindications become less meaningful. Certainly, the danger goes up if the neck is thick or if there is some bleeding tendency.

Traumatic tracheal injury with subcutaneous emphysema of the neck would render opening the airway above that point of questionable value. Lack of training would be a contraindication.

Precautions

Staying in the midline is a major precaution (Figures 3.18 and 3.19). The inferior portion of the cricothyroid membrane is the most avascular part. It is also farthest from the vocal cords, and is the preferred area. Following the curve of the needle or angling a straight needle at 45 degrees lessens the chance of perforating the soft back wall of the trachea (Figure 3.20).

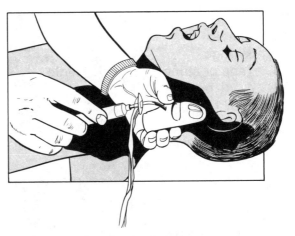

Figure 3–20   Goal of skill.

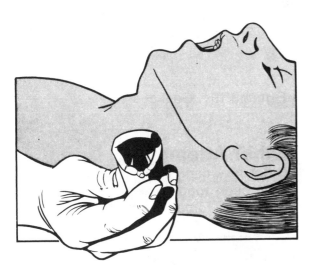

Figure 3–18   Top view of the larynx.

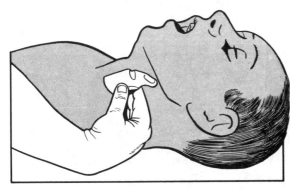

Figure 3–19   Side view of the larnyx.

Complications

Some complications of needle cricothyrostomy include false passage with mediastinal emphysema, bleeding, vocal cord damage, infection, and so forth. If the inhalation phase of ventilation with high-pressure oxygen exceeds 1 second, subcutaneous emphysema of the neck may quickly occur!

EQUIPMENT

Any No. 12 or No. 14 gauge catheter-over-needle can be introduced in this way through the cricothyroid membrane. One device, called the Omnicon Tracheostomy Kit, was developed as a curved needle particularly for this special procedure (Figure 3.21). A complete kit contains the following:

1. Iodine swab

2. Needle

3. Syringe

4. Tape or string to secure needle

5. A No. 3 pediatric endotracheal adapter with a 15-mm connection

6. High-flow oxygen source (50 psi) to release valve

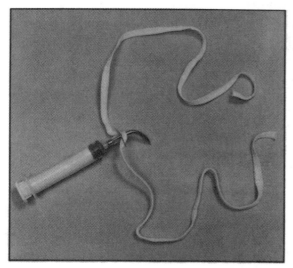

Figure 3-21 Needle cricothyrostomy kit.

SKILL SEQUENCE

Reassure the Patient

The paramedic should briefly explain the procedure to the patient if the patient is still awake.

Note Other Attempts

Other less dangerous maneuvers should have been tried first (Figure 3.22). Attempt

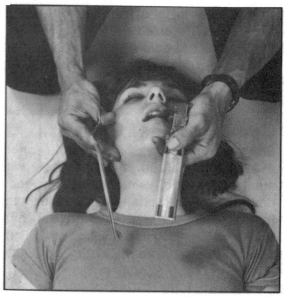

Figure 3-23 Attempt removal with Magill forceps.

with Magill forceps is indicated (Figure 3.23).

Palpate

A roll is placed under the back and neck (Figure 3.24). Then the cricothyroid membrane is palpated with the left hand, using the thyroid cartilage and cricoid cartilage as landmarks (Figure 3.25).

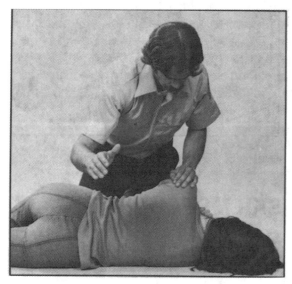

Figure 3-22 Basic maneuvers for foreign body.

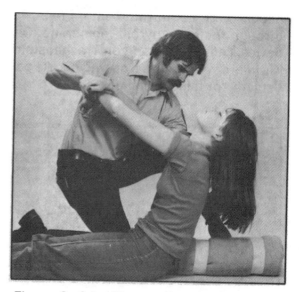

Figure 3-24 Place roll under back and neck.

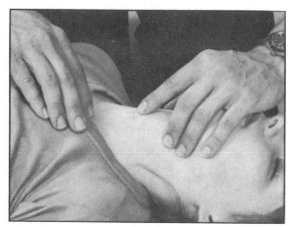

Figure 3-25   Palpate cricothyroid membrane.

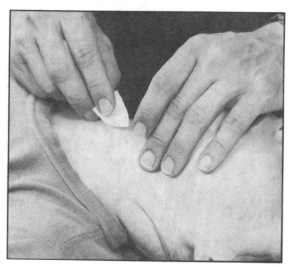

Figure 3-26   Prep neck.

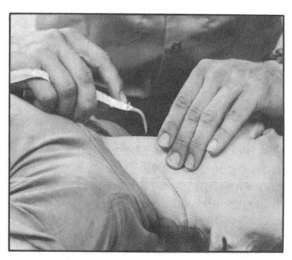

Figure 3-27   Insert needle through skin.

Prep

The area is prepped with iodine (Figure 3.26). A curved or straight needle is attached to a syringe and placed in the right hand. The needle is advanced through the lower half of the cricothyroid membrane (Figures 3.27 to 3.29).

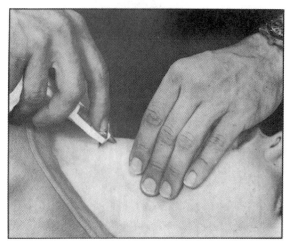

Figure 3-28   Begin needle rotation into trachea.

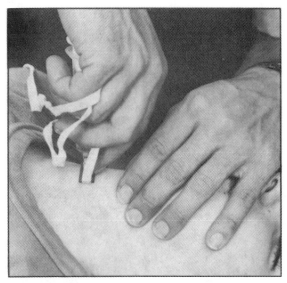

Figure 3-29   Complete rotation into trachea.

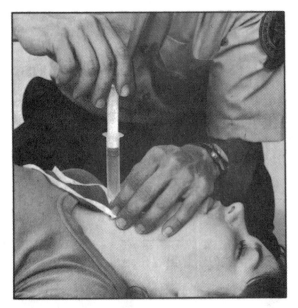

Figure 3–30   Aspirate syringe.

Aspirate

Air is aspirated *freely* or needle is removed (Figure 3.30).

Ventilate

The syringe plunger may be removed and one mouth-to-barrel ventilation may be tried (Figure 3.31).

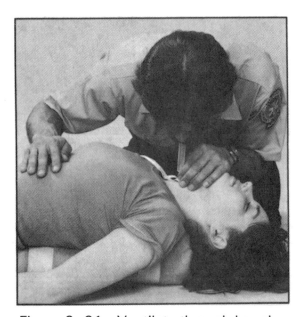

Figure 3–31   Ventilate through barrel.

Attach the Oxygen Source

The needle hub is connected to a No. 3 pediatric adapter. A 15-mm adapter end is connected to the oxygen source (Figure 3.32). Ventilation should cause the chest to rise. Do not exceed 1 second. Confirm position by listening to the chest. In case of sudden swelling of the neck, remove and replace. The correct oxygen source for insufflation is a jet of oxygen at 50 psi pressure rather than a demand valve (Figure 3.33)

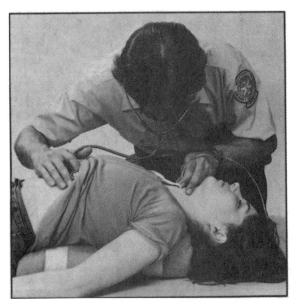

Figure 3–32   Ventilate using oxygen source.

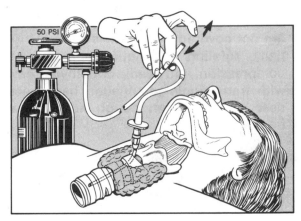

Figure 3–33   Oxygen jet.

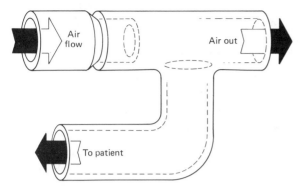

Figure 3–34 Detail of valve.

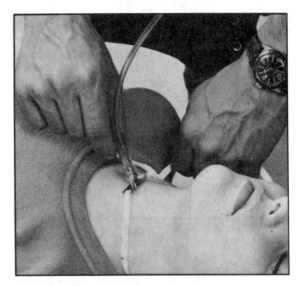

Figure 3–35 Secure in place.

The T-piece system shown in Figure 3.34 permits positive pressure when the oxygen flow is covered on negative pressure during exhalation. These pressures make up for the small needle size.

Secure

Secure in place by tying square knots on both sides (Figure 3.35).

LAB PRACTICE

The following Percutaneous Transtracheal Ventilation Procedure Guide is to be used during lab practice of this skill. Paired students take turns being rescuer and evaluator.

PERCUTANEOUS TRANSTRACHEAL VENTILATION PROCEDURE GUIDE

Rescuer's Name _____ Date _____ Evaluator _____

Directions for Evaluator: Place a check beside each item whenever an exam step is omitted, performed improperly, or presented improperly.

Step	Evaluation
1. Try basic maneuvers.	_____
2. Attempt removal with Magill forceps.	_____
3. Place roll under back and neck.	_____
4. Palpate cricothyroid membrane.	_____
5. Prep neck.	_____
6. Insert needle through skin.	_____
7. Rotate into trachea.	_____
8. Aspirate syringe.	_____
9. Ventilate through barrel.	_____
10. Ventilate using oxygen source.	_____
11. Secure in place.	_____
12. Connect to oxygen T-piece.	_____
13. Close "T" for 1-second inhalation.	_____
14. Open "T" for 4-second exhalation.	_____

SUMMARY

Most of the skills the paramedic will apply to breathing problems are found at the basic level—oxygen, positive pressure, and so forth. The next most common skill will be the use of drugs to treat pulmonary edema or bronchospasm. (These drugs are not discussed in this book.) Finally, rotating tourniquets, pleural decompression, and needle cricothyrostomy with transcricoid insufflation have been described here even though they may not be commonly used.

SKILL PROFICIENCY TESTING

Skill   Rotating Tourniquets (Venous Constriction Bands; Figure 3.36)

Performance   Demonstrate how to put on rotating tourniquets.

Conditions
1. Evaluator simulates a patient with pulmonary edema.
2. Base hospital has just confirmed an order for rotating tourniquets.
3. Four 1-inch Penrose Drains are visible among other equipment.
4. The evaluator has a simulated IV in the right arm.

Standard
1. Rescuer introduces himself or herself and offers reassurance. ☐
2. Rescuer places Penrose Drains around the proximal aspect of both thighs and the left arm. ☐
3. Tightness approximates that of IV tourniquet. ☐
4. Checks pulse after tourniquets are applied. ☐
5. Tourniquets applied within 1 minute. ☐

All criteria must be met to pass.

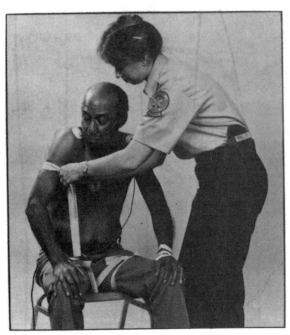

Figure 3–36

Student's Name _____ Date _____ Evaluator _____

Pass/Fail

SKILL PROFICIENCY TESTING

Skill Pleural Decompression (Needle Thoracostomy; Figure 3.37)

Performance Demonstrate how to decompress the pleura in a simulated case of tension pneumothorax using needle thoracostomy.

Conditions
1. Skeleton is placed on table in the supine position, with simulated chest skin cover.

2. Simulated patient has signs of tension pneumothorax.

3. Base hospital has given orders to use pleural decompression.

4. Equipment needed is large intercath, clean scissors, and iodine prep (dry but simulated).

Standard
1. Rescuer follows Needle Thoracostomy Procedure Guide, making no more than two errors. ☐

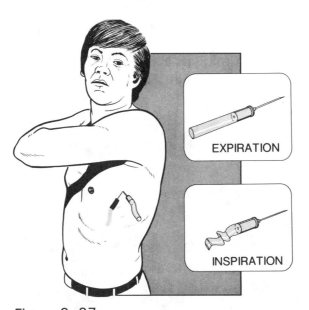

Figure 3–37

Student's Name _____ Date _____ Evaluator _____

Pass/Fail

SKILL PROFICIENCY TESTING

Skill Percutaneous Transtracheal Ventilation (Figure 3.38).

Performance Rescuer demonstrates how to perform percutaneous transtracheal ventilation.

Conditions
1. Larynx is simulated or an anesthetized dog is used.
2. Kit similar to Omnicon Tracheostomy Kit is available.
3. Pediatric 3.0-mm ET tube adapter and demand valve are available.
4. Rescuer is informed that manikin simulates patient with intractable complete airway obstruction, all manual maneuvers have been exhausted, and the base hospital has ordered a needle cricothyrostomy.

Standard
1. Rescuer follows Needle Cricothyrostomy Procedure Guide, making no more than two errors. ☐
2. Total limit: 60 seconds. ☐

All criteria must be met to pass.

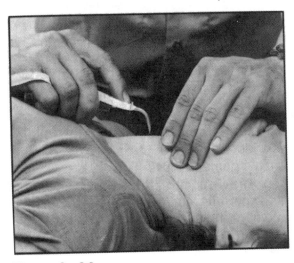

Figure 3-38

Student's Name _____ Date _____ Evaluator _____

Pass/Fail

4

Circulation Skills

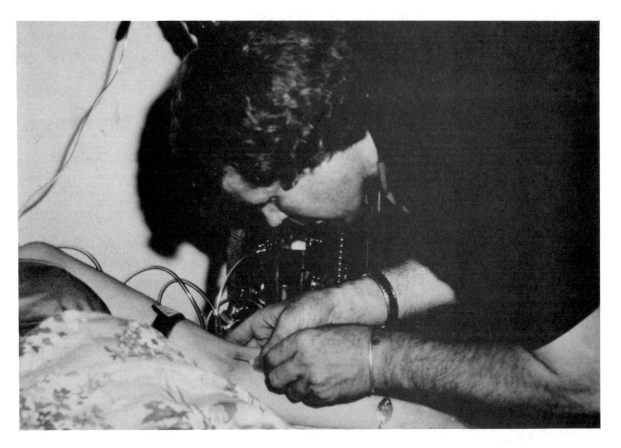

Skills Objectives

- **Antishock Trousers**—Demonstrate how to apply, maintain, and remove antishock trousers properly.

- **Trauma IV**—Demonstrate how to select and initiate a trauma IV on a simulated patient in shock.

Outline

Circulation Skills Description

Antishock Trousers
Trauma IV

Skill Proficiency Testing

Introduction
Special Considerations

Judgment
Equipment
Skill Sequence
Lab Practice

Circulation Skills Description
INTRODUCTION

Circulation is the third priority. The two priorities more important than circulation involve two aspects or respiration: airway—the passageway for air, and breathing—the mechanics of moving air. Circulation involves the perfusion of the body so that vital molecules (such as oxygen and glucose) get to the cells and wastes (such as carbon dioxide and metabolic acids) are removed from the cells.

For perfusion to take place, three components of the circulatory system must be working: the pump (the heart), the correct volume of fluid (blood), and the tone of the tubes (blood vessels). The partial loss of any one of these elements can lead to shock (poor perfusion of vital organs); the total loss of any element will lead to death.

SPECIAL CONSIDERATIONS
Patient Problems

The five common patient problems the rescuer faces in care of circulation are as follows: external bleeding, internal bleeding, shock, chest pain with risk of arrhythmia, and cardiac arrest. The four steps for the control of bleeding—direct pressure, elevation, pressure point, and tourniquet—are discussed in *Basic Life Support Skills Manual* for the EMT.

Cardiac dysrhythmias are discussed later in this book. Therefore, the main circulation problem being addressed at the advanced level in this chapter is the treatment of internal bleeding and/or shock. This same procedure applies to extensive external bleed in conjunction with BLS measures. The primary skills involve use of antishock trousers and a trauma (volume replacement) IV.

Types of Shock

Although shock can occur secondarily to loss of airway or impaired breathing, commonly it is a primary event. While many textbooks list 10 or 12 types of shock, the new paramedic texts are starting to emphasize four main categories: pump failure, pump obstruction, low volume (hypovolemia), and low resistance (distributive). Each of these can occur in either the traumatic situation or the nontraumatic, medical situation.

Antishock Trousers

For many years shock has been treated at the basic level of raising the legs to encourage increased return of blood from the veins of the legs. (Tipping the entire body so that the head is down has been discouraged because abdominal pressure on the diaphragm decreases inspiratory excursions.) Antishock trousers (Figure 4.1) accomplish the same goal more effectively. Originally, it was taught that the pressure suits squeeze some two units (about a quart) of blood out of the legs and abdomen and return it to the central circulation. More recently, published articles suggest that the real mechanism of the trousers is to increase peripheral or systemic vascular resistance (SVR) and thus increase blood pressure. This is the currently accepted theory of how it works. In either case, there is nearly universal agreement by emergency physicians that

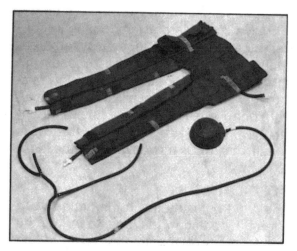

Figure 4–1 Antishock trousers.

the device is effective in the treatment of shock.

In Los Angeles, the trousers have also been advocated for the situation of massive trauma causing cardiopulmonary arrest (EMD), since the odds favor the hypothesis that massive internal hemorrhage has occurred. The application of the trousers is combined with fluid replacement and transport to a trauma center.

The antishock trousers are also considered a reasonable splint of the lower extremities or the pelvis, although with femur fractures they should be placed in combination with a traction splint. A number of physicians have published articles about the use of antishock trousers for such delicate situations as cardiogenic shock, where fluid challenge could be tried and yet is readily reversed (Table 4.1).

Table 4.1. TYPES OF SHOCK.

Category	Trauma	Medical
Cardiogenic	Pericardial tamponade	Cardiogenic shock
Hypovolemic	Bleeding spleen	Bleeding ulcer
Distributive	Spinal shock	Anaphylactic shock Septic shock
Obstructive	Pericardial tamponade Tension pneumothorax	Pulmonary embolus Aortic aneurysm

In 1980, the Advanced Trauma Life Support courses of the American College of Surgeons was initiated. The alternative term *antishock garment* (ASG) was introduced. Both names are used currently.

JUDGMENT

Indications

Antishock trousers are indicated for hypovolemic shock (especially for bleeding below the diaphragm) or distributive shock. They are recommended if the systolic blood pressure is 80 mm Hg or lower; 100 mm Hg if other obvious signs of shock are present.

They may be used for distributive shock, for temporary venous volume increase in order to get an IV started, or for continuous abdominal pressure. They are warranted in such abdominal emergencies as a gunshot wound to the abdomen or a leaking aortic aneurysm.

Antishock trousers have been suggested for cardiopulmonary arrest from trauma where there is high probability of massive internal or external hemorrhage. They have applications for leg splinting but should be used with a traction splint on a midshaft femur fracture.

Contraindications

Antishock trousers are used cautiously in bleeding above the diaphragm since the possibility of increasing the bleeding as the blood pressure comes up must be considered. Many experienced physicians no longer consider bleeding scalp, possible subdural hematoma, tension pneumothorax, and pericardial tamponade as contraindications for antishock trousers, reasoning that in many of these cases the shock can be improved temporarily by raising the venous pressure above normal. Pulmonary edema is an absolute contraindication, since it would almost always worsen as fluid is moved up from the legs.

Precautions

One must be cautious, in the patient with arterial bleeding in the legs, to inflate the suit to top pressures to avoid bleeding under the suit. The paramedic must also remember that blood flow to the kidneys will probably be reduced with this device, and long-term application should be discouraged. Urination and defecations may rarely occur, but this should not discourage its use.

In uterine pregnancy, the abdominal compartment should not be inflated. In tubal pregnancy with bleeding it may be inflated.

Complications

Sudden removal of antishock trousers in the emergency department may lead to profound shock. Gradual removal of (deflate half the chambers) 5 mm Hg of suit pressure at a time, *rechecking blood pressure,* releasing from the abdominal compartment first, may prevent this complication. At least one large bore IV should be in place, and substantial fluid replacement given, before removal. Sometimes the device is removed only when the surgeon is ready and the patient is in the operating room.

Increasing a hemothorax would also be a potential hazard. Overinflation, with decreased profusion to the kidneys or legs, can lead to obvious complications. Arterial bleeding under the trousers can occur.

EQUIPMENT

The main brands of antishock trousers have either pressure dials or safety release valves to determine tightness (Figures 4.2 and 4.3). The dials indicate that above 30 mm Hg is a danger zone, but most of the time much higher pressures are needed—up to the maximum 100 mm Hg. The brands with a safety release valve release air at about 104 mm Hg. The best approach is to inflate either suit to the point of *clinical improve-*

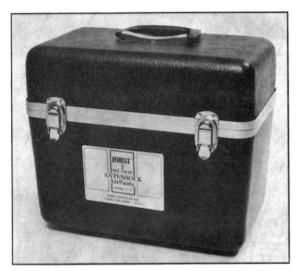

Figure 4-2   Case.

cessively in the leg compartment of an adult suit, and infants in the leg of a pediatric suit. The skill sequence will cover the multiple-dial system first and then the Velcro safety valve type of suit.

Prefolding the antishock trousers is important so that upon rapid removal from the case the orientation of the suit is clear. It is very frustrating and embarrassing to try to figure out under pressure which is the proper side up or which leg compartment is right. Each paramedic company should standardize the folding of the suits, including use of tape to maintain necessary folds. Also, open placement of antishock trousers on a gurney when responding to obvious trauma saves considerable time in application.

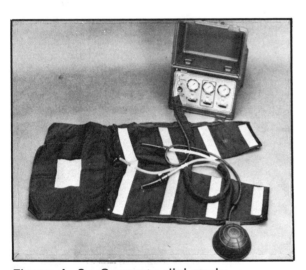

Figure 4-3   Separate dial pack.

SKILL SEQUENCE—

Introduce Self

Paramedic begins with introduction and reassurance. The paramedic recognizes hypovolemic shock from bleeding, through subjective history, general pale appearance, low blood pressure, fast pulse, and so forth. He follows protocol or confirms use with base hospital.

Perform a Preassessment

Foot pulses, sensation, and motor function in both legs are checked as part of patient evaluation. Asucultate lungs for signs of pulmonary edema.

ment. Always remember to look at your patient's physiological response.

Some brands offer Velcro or zipper closures. The Velcro is faster and thus more popular, but can become less effective after numerous machine washings. Clear suits allow visual patient examinations even with the suit on.

There are a variety of sizes, from extra-large adult to pediatric. Some paramedics have reported treating small children suc-

Prepare the Suit

Prefolded suit is opened to proper position (Figure 4.4) and is then brought up between legs to perineum as patient's legs are lifted (Figure 4.5). Patient is centered (Figure 4.6). Leg compartments are extended over patient (Figure 4.7) and then closed (Figure 4.8).

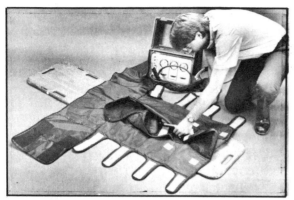

Figure 4-4   Prepare pants for patient by prefolding.

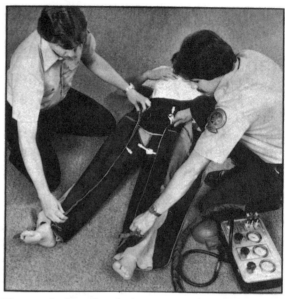

Figure 4-7   Extend pants over patient.

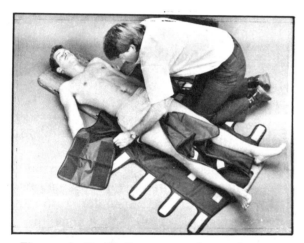

Figure 4-5   Pull pants under patient.

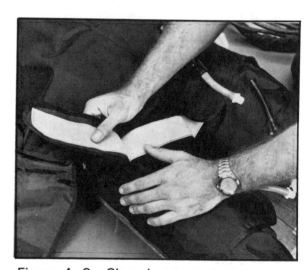

Figure 4-8   Close leg compartments.

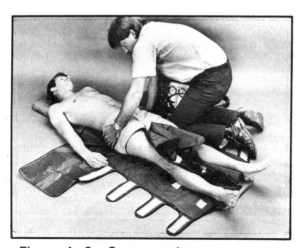

Figure 4-6   Center patient.

Secure the Abdominal Compartment

The abdominal belt is tightened to prevent ballooning during inflation. (Figure 4.9).

Connect the Air Tubes

Air tubes are connected to antishock trouser connectors (Figure 4.10).

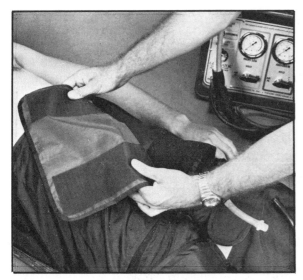

Figure 4–9   Tighten abdominal compartment.

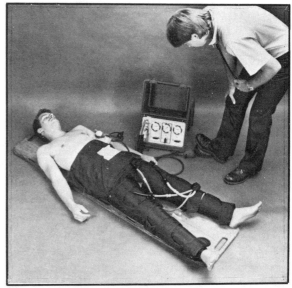

Figure 4–11   Inflate legs.

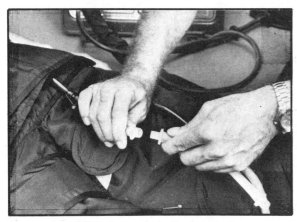

Figure 4–10   Attach inflation tubes.

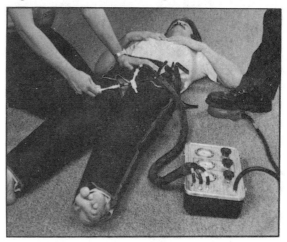

Figure 4–12   Inflate abdominal compartment.

Inflate the Suit

Leg compartments are filled to at least 50 mm Hg (30 mm Hg is usually too low) on the dials with the dials in the "Air In" position; the patient's blood pressure is rechecked and if satisfactory, the dials are then turned to "Hold" (Figure 4.11). The abdominal compartment is similarly filled (Figure 4.12). Afterward, foot pulses are rechecked (Figure 4.13).

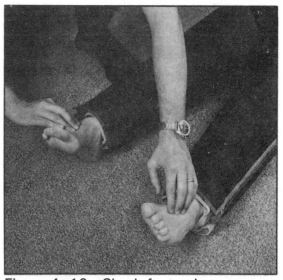

Figure 4–13   Check foot pulses.

Recheck Vitals

Vital signs are rechecked; the suit pressure is increased to 100 mm Hg if needed. Often a paramedic will start one or two IVs at this point.

Deflate Slowly

Although rarely done in the field, the technique for deflation should also be learned. If fluid volume is restored and blood pressure is normal, deflation should be tried slowly using the abdominal compartment first—5 mm Hg at a time, watching blood pressure as described earlier and adding fluids as needed.

The valves on the tubing of the suit with gauges must be open during filling. While they can be closed during transport, the gauges will not then reflect the effective pressures. Unless transport terrain is very rough, the tubing valves should be left open during transport so that any drop in suit pressure an be recognized early.

LAB PRACTICE

The following Antishock Trousers Procedure Guide is to be used during lab practice of this skill. Paired students take turns being rescuer and evaluator.

Trauma IV

There are generally two types of intravenous setups that should be used in the prehospital setting: a trauma IV to replace fluid volume and a medical IV used as a pathway or IV lifeline into the bloodstream for rapid administration of medications. In dealing with most types of shock, the trauma IV is indicated and is discussed in this chapter. For a general comparison of the equipment used, a list is supplied in Table 4.2.

It is clear from the list in Table 4.2 that the goal of the trauma IV is to get the Ringer's lactate, or normal saline, into the bloodstream rapidly to replace lost fluid or blood. Normal saline is a satisfactory alternative to Ringer's lactate and preferred by many.

Blood Replacement

Blood consists primarily of water with dissolved salt and glucose, protein particles in suspension, and various blood cells. In the prehospital setting blood is seldom available, and a temporary substitute must be given.

Table 4.2. EQUIPMENT FOR TRAUMA AND MEDICAL IVs.

	Trauma IV	Medical IV
Typical solution	1000 cc Ringer's lactate or normal saline	500 ml dextrose 5% in water
Typical tubing	Macrodrip chamber— fast flow	Microdrip chamber—slow flow
Extension tubing	Same	Same
Catheter-over-needle	Large—size No. 14	Small—size No. 20
Method of taping catheter	Same	Same

ANTISHOCK TROUSERS PROCEDURE GUIDE

Rescuer's Name_____ Date_____ Evaluator_____

Directions for Evaluator: Place a check beside each item whenever an exam step is omitted, performed improperly, or presented improperly.

Step	Method	Evaluation
1. Introduce self	a. Introduce self and reassure.	_____
	b. Confirm presence of shock.	_____
	c. Secure permission from base.	
2. Preassess	a. Evaluate circulation, include check of lung sound to R/O pulmonary edema.	_____
3. Prepare the suit	a. Open case or bag.	_____
	b. Open suit.	_____
	c. Pull under patient.	_____
	d. Center patient.	_____
	e. Extend suit over patient.	_____
4. Secure the compartments	a. Close leg compartments.	_____
	b. Close abdominal area.	_____
5. Connect the air tubes	a. Connect three air valves.	_____
6. Fill the suit	a. Inflate leg compartments.	_____
	b. Then inflate abdominal area.	_____
	c. Bring gauges to 100 mm Hg (or instructor's preference).	_____
	d. Turn gauges to hold.	_____
	e. Inflate until safety valve hisses.*	_____
	f. Recheck foot pulses.	_____
	g. Recheck vital signs.	_____
7. Deflate slowly	a. Deflate slowly.	_____
	b. Deflate abdominal compartment first.	_____

*Some instructors have students close valves and even tape them in the closed position at this point, to avoid leakage during transport.

The most common solution used in trauma is Ringer's lactate, a solution of sodium glucose, and other electrolytes in water.

The most important difference between blood and Ringer's lactate is that the latter lacks red blood cells to carry oxygen. Thus Ringer's lactate supports the fluid volume problem in shock but does not restore the oxygen-carrying capacity that has been lost. It can substitute in a healthy person for up to almost two-thirds of blood loss before life systems will begin to fail.

The rule of fluid replacement, published in 1980 by the American College of Surgeons, is to give Ringer's lactate three times the volume of blood loss. Often it is unclear if extra fluid volume will be helpful. In this case often 200 ml of salt solution (Ringer's lactate or saline) is run in and the patient is examined for effect. This is called a fluid challenge.

JUDGMENT

Indications

A trauma IV is indicated whenever rapid restoration of blood volume is, or may be needed in the prehospital setting. Often an IV is begun on any traumatized patient as a precaution, in case bleeding suddenly occurs internally. Although the word "trauma" is emphasized, the trauma IV is also indicated for such non-trauma situations as a bleeding duodenal ulcer, dehydrated diabetic, or bleeding tubal pregnancy.

Contraindications

Because the solutions used for IV therapy in trauma expand the blood volume effectively, they also set up the risk of fluid overload. The overload usually shows up as pulmonary edema presenting as shortness of breath combined with the objective finding of rales at both lung bases. The main contraindication with this type of IV is pulmonary edema. Obviously, the combined conditions of pulmonary edema and shock,

common in cardiogenic shock, requires very delicate treatment.

Precautions

Because of the risk of overload, it is a good habit in general to follow both the blood pressure and the breath sounds when rapidly administering fluids. There are certain precautions to using any medication by vein: (1) make sure that the fluid is clear rather than cloudy; (2) do not contaminate the bag or tubing (use of teeth to open packages must be discouraged); (3) check expiration date; and (4) try to avoid air bubbles.

Another precaution is a consideration of whether or not to wear gloves. This is a systems choice focusing on the potential risk of contracting a disease such as AIDS. The time of greatest risk is recapping needles where gloves do not protect self puncture.

Complications

The potential complications of IV therapy are many, which is why it is not a part of basic life support training. When the techniques are taught carefully, the complication rate need not be high.

LOCAL. Local complications include the following:

1. *Pain*—at needle site due to skin pressure, tissue invasion, and/or infiltration of fluid outside the vein

2. *Infection*—usually not noticed until several days after the IV placement but related to sterility of original techniques

3. *Nerve or artery damage*—related to IVs placed near surface arteries or nerves

4. *Tissue sloughing*—many occur when certain drugs, such as adrenaline or calcium, are used with an infiltrated IV

5. *Pneumothorax*—possible with certain central vein techniques

6. *Intra-aterial injection*—inadvertent placement of an IV in an artery, which can lead to dry gangrene if irritating medications are added

SYSTEMIC. Systemic complications include the following:

1. *Fainting*—This may be due to emotional reaction to needles.

2. *Systemic infection*—This can result from contaminated solutions (IV solutions must be clear!).

3. *Air embolism*—IVs placed in large veins, such as the subclavian, may suck air in rather than bleed back when disconnected, thus sending air into the heart or lungs.

4. *Anaphylaxis*—Generally this is due to medications added rather than the IV solution itself.

5. *Pulmonary edema*—IV solutions containing sodium chloride, such as Ringer's lactate, can add so much fluid that they overload patient and lead to pulmonary edema.

6. *Catheter embolization*—It is possible to have the plastic catheter sheer off and travel into the heart or lungs. **A plastic catheter should never be retracted through or over a needle.**

7. *Pulmonary thromboembolism*—IVs left in the legs, particularly for several days, can lead to deep vein thrombosis and embolism to the lungs. This is not an initial concern in prehospital care.

EQUIPMENT

The following equipment would be advisable in starting a trauma IV: a 1000-ml bag of Ringer's lactate, macrodrip tubing, extension tubing, large catheter-over-needle, venous constriction band, alcohol swab, iodine

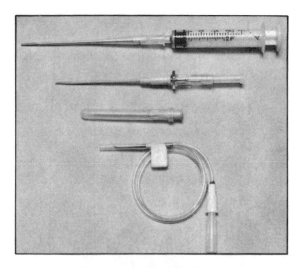

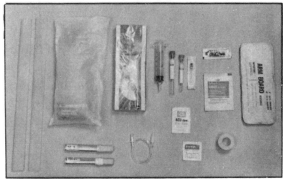

Figure 4–14   Trauma IV kit and needle types.

swab, 2 × 2 gauze, 1-inch tape, and an arm board. This equipment can be packaged into a kit (Figure 4.14).

Vein Choice
Peripheral Veins

Peripheral vein sites include the entire arm, ankle, or foot, and external jugular in the neck (Figures 4.15 to 4.18). The scalp is an optional site in the newborn child. The preferred peripheral sites for IV insertion are as follows: dorsal hand, dorsal forearm, upper arm, and the anticubital fossa or elbow crease. The upper arm, although rarely taught, is particularly helpful in the patient who is combative or having seizures. The left hand is preferred over the right because

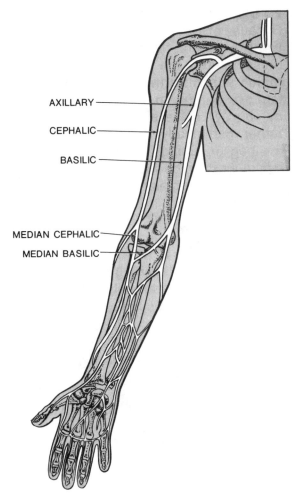

Figure 4-15 Upper extremity veins.

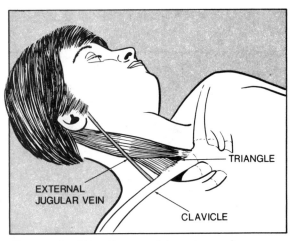

Figure 4-17 External jugular vein.

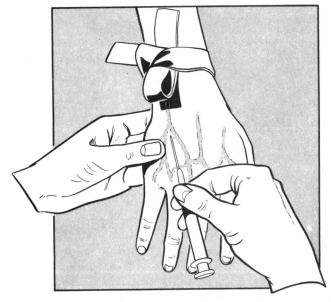

Figure 4-16 Back-of-hand veins.

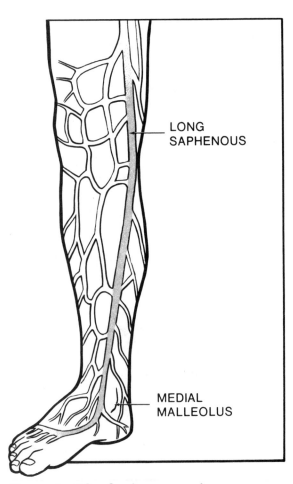

Figure 4-18 Saphenous vein.

of ease of maintenance in the ambulance and comfort over the first few days of hospitalization.

Central veins, which are occasionally used when peripheral veins are absent or unavailable, include the internal jugular, subclavian, and femoral veins. The femoral vein is the preferred vein of the three during a cardiac arrest situation because it least interferes with CPR.

SKILL SEQUENCE (PERIPHERAL VEIN)

Confirm the Order

Upon receipt of the order, paramedics must confirm whether or not the order is consistent with their training. If so, they confirm the order stating the base hospital, rescue unit number, and the IV skill requested:

> John Muir Base, this is Pomeroy Paramedic Unit 82 confirming the order to administer IV Ringer's lactate, wide open to a stable BP.

Preparing the IV

The paramedic must be able to recognize the equipment common to all IVs as well as those specially suited for the trauma IV.

The IV bag is in a plastic envelope that is torn open easily if the tear notch is located (Figure 4.19). The bag should be checked for cloudiness and then squeezed for leaks. The name of the solution is read once (Figure 4.20). The expiration date is checked. The IV tubing and extention tubing are opened and connected in sterile fashion (Figure 4.21).

The control valve below the drip chamber is closed (Figure 4.22) and the IV tubing is inserted into the inverted IV solution bag (Figure 4.23). The IV solution may be handed to an assistant or a bystander, who is told to keep it at about shoulder height. Next, the drip chamber is squeezed until it is half full of solution (Figure 4.24).

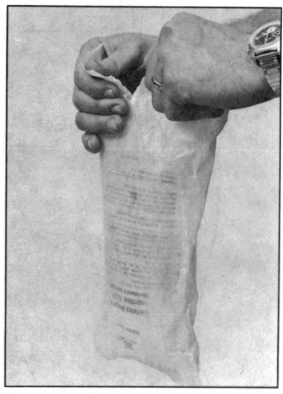

Figure 4–19   Tear the envelope bag.

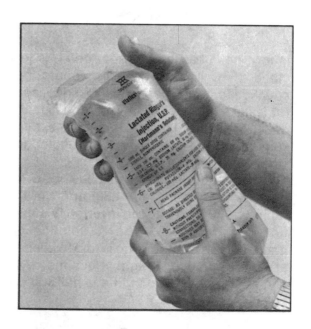

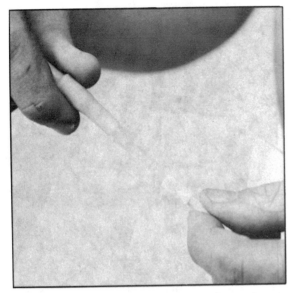

Figure 4-21   Connect extension tubing.

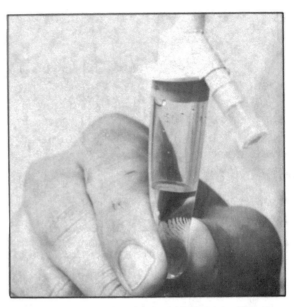

Figure 4-24   Fill drip chamber halfway.

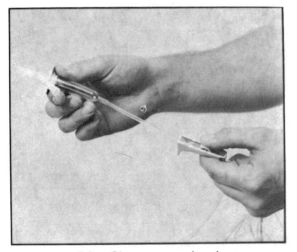

Figure 4-22   Close control valve.

At this point the extension tubing tip is uncapped (Figure 4.25) and the cap is held in the fingers so as not to contaminate. The tubing valves are opened so that IV fluid will fill the main tubing and the extension tubing (Figure 4.26). Excess fluid is allowed to drip in the IV envelope so that the floor does not get wet (Figure 4.27). Then the tubing valve is closed (Figure 4.28) and the extension tubing is recapped (Figure 4.29).

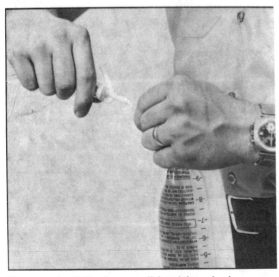

Figure 4-23   Insert IV tubing in bag.

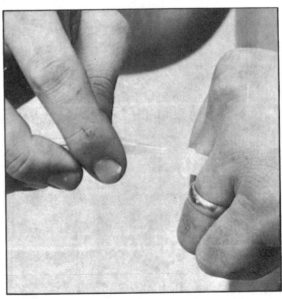

Figure 4-25   Uncap extension tubing.

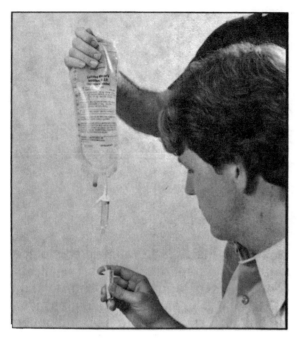

Figure 4-26 Open control valve.

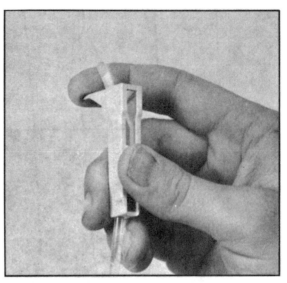

Figure 4-28 Close valve.

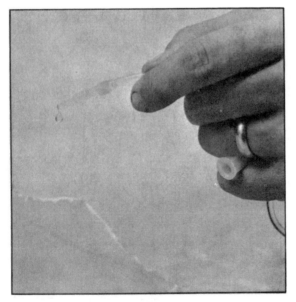

Figure 4-27 Fill IV line.

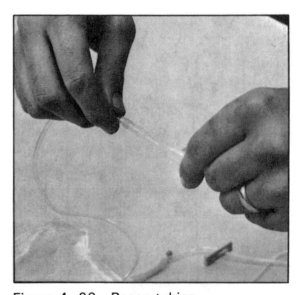

Figure 4-29 Recap tubing.

Insert the IV

The venous constriction band or "tourniquet" (rubber or Velcro) is placed around the patient's upper arm just tight enough to occlude venous return (Figures 4.30 to 4.33). A blood pressure cuff pumped up works well too.

The paramedic explains that he or she is going to start an IV to help the patient. The patient can refuse if mentally competent. If the patient agrees, the paramedic palpates the veins of the forearm (Figure 4.34) and tears strips of tape for use later (Figure 4.35).

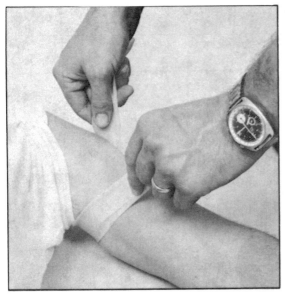

Figure 4–30   Encircle arm with constriction band.

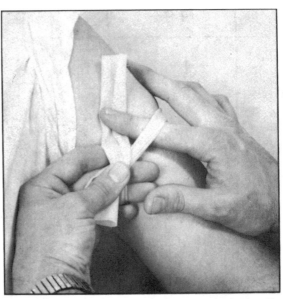

Figure 4–32   Reach under to produce slip knot.

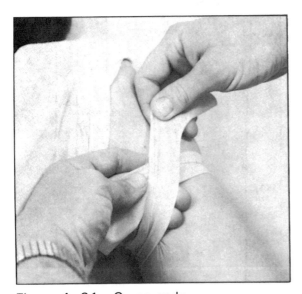

Figure 4–31   Cross ends.

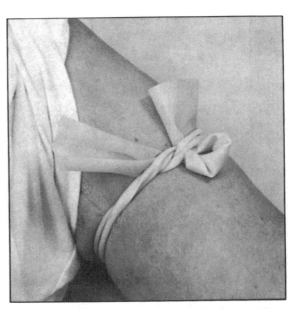

Figure 4–33   Complete band placement.

The skin is cleansed with an iodine swab in increasing sized concentric circles (Figure 4.36). Following this with an alcohol swab (Figure 4.37) prevents later iodine reactions. The vein is then stabilized with the paramedic's thumb. The skin is entered at (Figure 4.38) 30 to 45 degrees at the side of the vein (some prefer entering directly above the vein), with the bevel of the needle facing upward. The vein is entered

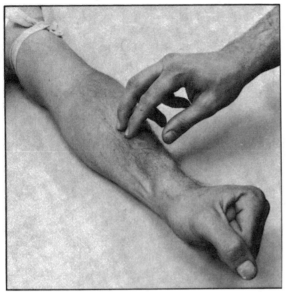

Figure 4–34   Palpate vein.

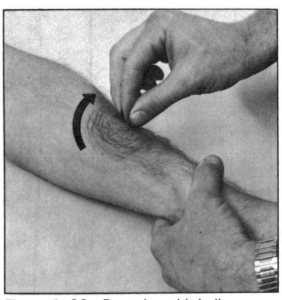

Figure 4–36   Prep site with iodine.

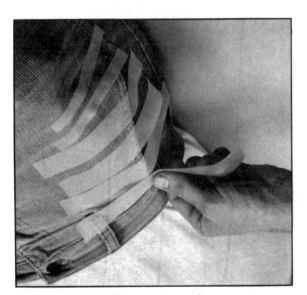

Figure 4–35   Tear strips of tape.

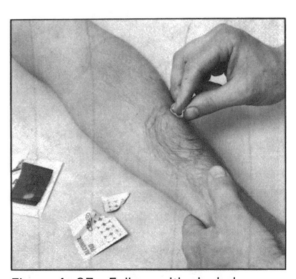

Figure 4–37   Follow with alcohol.

(Figure 4.39) and if there is blood return, the catheter is advanced over the needle (Figure 4.40). Once this occurs, the catheter is never pulled back over the needle as this might cause shearing. Blood samples are taken (Figure 4.41) with a syringe of size 10 cc or greater, and the constricting band is removed (Figure 4.42).

The paramedic can avoid getting blood around the site by compressing the entered

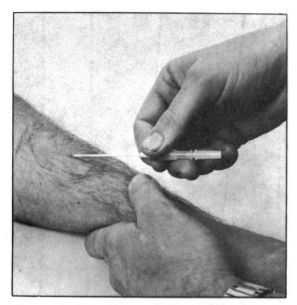

Figure 4-38   Enter skin.

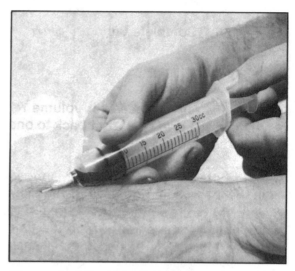

Figure 4-41   Take blood sample.

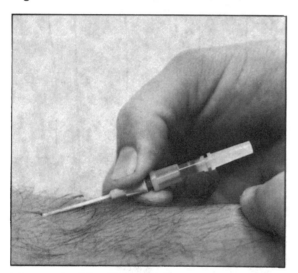

Figure 4-39   Enter vein.

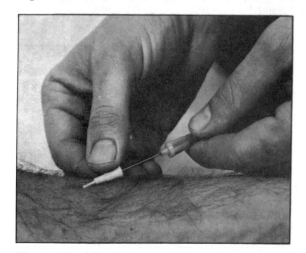

Figure 4-40   Advance IV catheter.

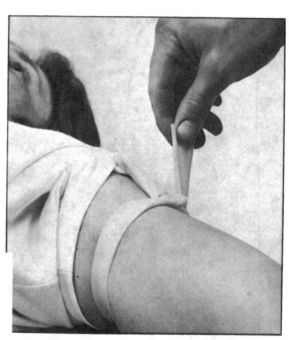

Figure 4-42   Release band (tourniquet).

vein near the tip of the catheter while connecting the extension tubing. The IV extension tubing is connected to the catheter (Figure 4.43), and the IV clamp is opened (Figure 4.44) to assure free flow. Unless there is current need for volume replacement, the drip rate is set back to 1 drop per second.

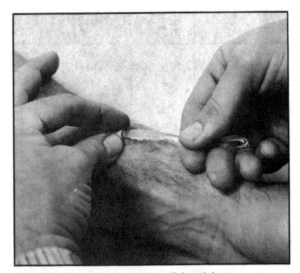

Figure 4-43 Connect IV tubing.

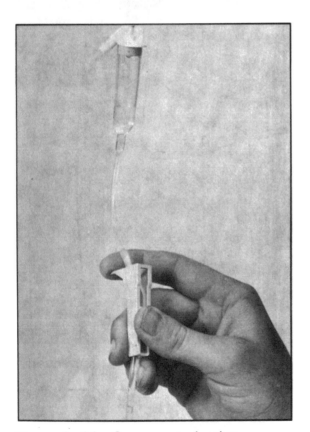

Figure 4-44 Open control valve.

Secure the IV

The 2 × 2 gauze is taped down over the insertion area of the skin. Placing antibiotic ointment at the insertion site is optional depending on the time available (Figure

4.45). The IV catheter is then secured with a loop of ½-inch tape torn from the 1-inch roll (Figure 4.46). The extension tubing is then looped back and secured with another piece of tape (Figure 4.47). The IV portals for drug administration must not be covered. The IV drip rate is then set precisely (Figure 4.48). Blood tubes may now be filled (Figure 4.49).

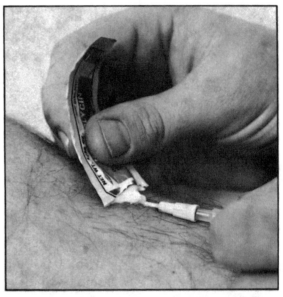

Figure 4-45 Apply antibacterial ointment.

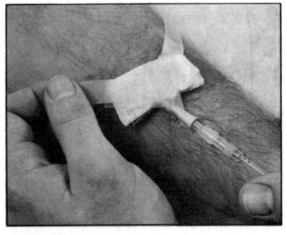

Figure 4-46 Secure 2 × 2 gauze and catheter.

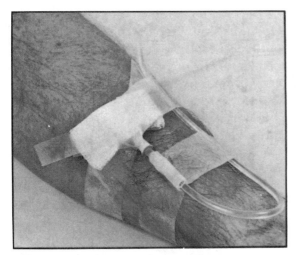

Figure 4–47   Complete taping.

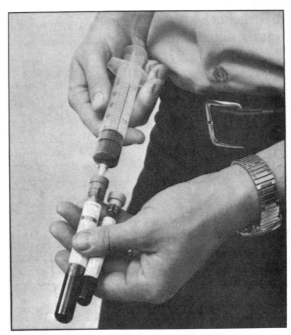

Figure 4–49   Fill blood tube containers.

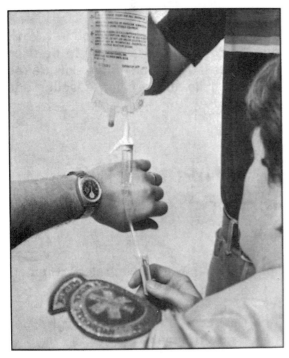

Figure 4–48   Time drip flow.

Troubleshoot the IV

The skill of IV insertion is not really understood well unless the paramedic is able to troubleshoot an IV that is not working well. The following steps systematically take the paramedic from the patient's arm back to the IV solution.

1.   Make sure that the tourniquet is off (often hidden under a shirt sleeve).

2.   Check the IV insertion site for swelling.

3.   Check the tubing valves to make sure that they are open.

4.   If the drip chamber is full, squeeze back half into the IV bag while it is temporarily inverted.

5.   Lower the bag below the IV insertion site and look for free blood return into the IV tubing.

6.   Gently compress the IV bag.

7.   Close the drip chamber valve and wrap the tubing around a penlight to compress it.

8.   Reopen the IV valve to see if the flow has been improved.

A poor IV is worse than no IV and should be replaced.

Confirm the IV Insertion

The paramedic should then get back on the radio or telephone and confirm that the IV has been started. The communication should include the base hospital, rescue unit name and number, IV skill completed, number of attempts, and change in patient if any:

> John Muir Base, this is Pomeroy 82 confirming the insertion of a trauma IV on the second attempt. After 200 ml of fluid, the palpable blood pressure has come up from 40 to 50.

LAB PRACTICE

The following Detailed Peripheral Venipuncture Procedure Guide is to be used during lab practice of this skill. Paired students take turns being rescuer and evaluator.

Central Vein Cannulation

The main purpose for being able to cannulate a central vein in the field is as a backup when peripheral veins are unavailable. The two most common approaches are the femoral vein and the subclavian vein. The femoral vein is best during cardiac arrest since it avoids extra crowding around the upper body. The subclavian might be best in trauma where it will not get in the way of the antishock trousers often applied first. Both are extraordinary procedures and must be discussed with the local medical community before instituting. As with all difficult procedures done rarely, the real challenge is not teaching the skill the first time but keeping the skill up with continuing education. In this regard it is unfortunate that manikins for these procedures have not been developed. The internal jugular vein is a third central vein increasingly used.

The inclusion of these techniques in this manual does not imply the author's blanket endorsement of their prehospital use. The author does recognize that paramedics in some systems have been taught these procedures. They are mentioned for these paramedic systems. The real issues to be discussed concerning any extraordinary skills are as follows:

- Does the local law allow the skill?

- Do the physicians want the skill used in the prehospital setting?

- Can the skill be taught?

- Can the skill be maintained?

When these questions can be answered affirmatively medical control is maintained.

JUDGMENT

Indications

Central veins in the prehospital setting should only be sought when an IV is needed, peripheral veins are unavailable, the hospital base station has okayed the skill despite the delay it may cause, and the system in which the rescuer is working both teaches and allows the skill.

Contraindications

An extraordinary skill must be used only for extraordinary situations. A patient in cardiac arrest and more than 20 minutes from a hospital should probably have stabilization attempts even to an extraordinary degree rather than using moving CPR since survival will depend on some improvement in the field prior to transport. It would probably be contraindicated in a patient several minutes from a hospital regardless of the condition. Injuries near the IV sites would be contraindications as well, although IVs occasionally must be started through burned tissue.

DETAILED PERIPHERAL VENIPUNCTURE
PROCEDURE GUIDE

Rescuer's Name_____ Date_____ Evaluator_____

Directions for Evaluator: Place a check beside each item whenever an exam step is omitted, performed improperly, or presented improperly.

Sample Patient Problem:

1. Patient with hypotension from hypovolemia needing a trauma IV

2. IV manikin arm simulating patient arm

3. Evaluator acts as simulated base hospital to give orders, then later as bystander

4. Assorted IV equipment available for trauma IV and medical IV

Step   **Evaluation**

Confirming the Order

Paramedic evaluates whether or not the order is consistent with training, and if so, confirms the order stating base hospital, rescue unit number, and IV skill requested.

Evaluator reconfirms.

Preparing the IV

1. The paramedic correctly assembles the components of a trauma IV kit.
   a. 1000 ml of Ringer's lactate   _____
   b. Macrodrip tubing   _____
   c. Extension tubing   _____
   d. No. 16 or No. 14 needle   _____
   e. Venous tourniquet   _____
   f. Iodine swab and alcohol prep   _____
   g. 2 × 2 gauze pad   _____
   h. 1-inch tape   _____
   i. Arm board   _____

2. Opens IV bag envelope at the edge where it is notched.   _____

3. Examines IV bag for cloudiness and squeezes to check for leaks. _____

4. Reads name of the solution, checks expiration date.   _____

5. Opens IV tubing and extension tubing and connects.   _____

6. Closes control valve below the drip chamber.   _____

7. Inserts IV tubing in the IV solution bag portal.   _____

DETAILED PERIPHERAL VENIPUNCTURE
PROCEDURE GUIDE (Continued)

Rescuer's Name_____ Date_____ Evaluator_____

Step   **Evaluation**

8. Squeezes drip chamber until half full of solution. _____

9. Hands IV solution to the evaluator as a bystander. _____

10. Uncaps extension tubing: cap is held so that it will not become contaminated. _____

11. Opens IV tubing valve to allow the solution to flow through into the bag envelope until all bubbles are out of the tube. _____

12. Closes tubing valve and recaps extension tubing. _____

Inserting the IV

1. Places a constriction band around the patient's left arm just below the shoulder. _____

2. Explains that an IV is going to be started to make the patient feel better. _____

3. Palpates veins for resillience. _____

4. Cleanses skin with the iodine swab in concentric circles of increasing size and follows with an alcohol sponge. _____

5. Stabilizes vein distally with the rescuer's thumb. _____

6. Enters skin to the side of the vein at 30 to 45 degrees with the bevel of the needle facing upward. _____

7. Enters vein, obtains flashback, and advances the catheter of the catheter-over-needle. _____

8. Takes blood sample. _____

9. Removes constricting band. _____

10. Compresses the vein near the proximal tip of the catheter to prevent blood loss temporarily. _____

11. Connects IV extension tubing to the catheter. _____

12. Opens the IV clamp to assure free flow. _____

Securing the IV

1. Tapes 2 × 2 gauze and antibiotic ointment down over the insertion area of the skin. _____

2. Secures IV catheter next with a loop of ½-inch tape torn from the 1-inch roll. _____

DETAILED PERIPHERAL VENIPUNCTURE
PROCEDURE GUIDE (Continued)

Rescuer's Name_____ Date_____ Evaluator_____

Step   **Evaluation**

3. Loops extension tubing back and secures with another piece of tape.   _____

4. Does not cover IV portals.   _____

5. Rechecks IV drip rate to make sure that it has not changed from one drip per second.   _____

6. Fills blood tubes.   _____

Troubleshooting the IV
The evaluator explains that the IV is not working well and should be thoroughly checked.

1. Makes sure that the tourniquet is off.   _____

2. Checks IV insertion site for swelling.   _____

3. Checks IV tubing for valve closure.   _____

4. Checks drip chamber to make sure that it is half full.   _____

5. Gently compresses the IV bag if all these factors are present.   _____

6. Lowers bag and looks for blood return.   _____

7. Closes IV valve below drip chamber and wraps tubing around penlight, compressing it toward patient.   _____

8. Reopens IV valve to see if flow has improved.   _____

Confirming IV Insertion
Rescuer confirms that an IV has been started, including in communication the following:

1. Base hospital   _____

2. Rescue unit name and number   _____

3. IV skill completed   _____

4. Number of attempts   _____

5. Change in patient if any   _____

Total limit: 5 minutes

Precautions

For proper placement of central lines in the subclavian or jugular vein, the patient must be tipped with head down Trendelenburg position or antishock trousers are used to fill those veins. If this is not done, the incidence of complications goes up as the veins are harder to cannulate. Securing of the IV tubing once successfully in place is very important as air embolism with tubing separation can be rapid and lethal.

Complications

All of the usual complications of IV therapy are possible—infection, arterial puncture, pain, and so on. Air embolism is a special risk as mentioned above. Pneumothorax is common with the subclavian approach as the top of the lung lies close to the clavicle. The femoral vein cannulation probably has the lowest complication rate and might be the safest central vein field route. Other subclavian vein complications include hydrothorax (IV fluid in the pleural cavity), thoracic duct perforation (left side of neck—thus right side preferred), catheter embolism, arterial puncture, brachial plexus injury, vagus nerve injury, and so forth. Thoracotomies have occasionally been needed to repair damage to subclavian arteries.

EQUIPMENT

It is generally true that central veins require a catheter-over-needle at least 6 to 7 cm long as the vein may be 5 cm from the point of skin entry. This is more true of the subclavian vein than the femoral vein but the principle is good. Many types of central vein kits exist, but in the prehospital system the simple catheter-over-needle is recommended.

ANATOMICAL EMPHASIS

The central vein techniques involve cannulation of veins that are not visible from the surface. Therefore, they require a much greater appreciation of anatomy. Such anatomical or structural details also help the paramedic avoid complications as much as possible. Each of the three central vein approaches will be discussed—in terms of anatomy, diagram, advantages, disadvantages, technique steps, and lab practice—using the procedure guides.

Femoral Vein

A. ANATOMY.   The femoral vein lies consistently medial to the femoral artery as they cross below the inguinal ligament (Figure 4.50). Actually, five structures line up below the ligament, moving from lateral to medial: the femoral nerve, femoral artery, femoral vein, empty space, and lacuner ligament. This gives rise to the memory aid NAVEL. The key to the location of the femoral vein, then, is the femoral artery.

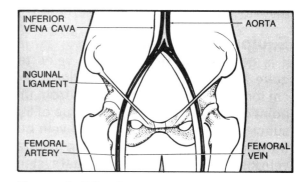

Figure 4–50   Anatomy of femoral vein.

The femoral artery is determined by two methods: (1) by estimating that the location is the midpoint between the symphysis pubis and the anterior iliac spine, and (2) actual palpation of the artery during a spontaneous or artificial pulse. The latter method is more accurate. The exact direction of the artery can be determined if it is felt by two fingers simultaneously.

B. ADVANTAGES

1.   Available even when peripheral veins are flat.

2. Does not interrupt CPR.

3. Rapid drug effect.

4. Patient does not need to be positioned in Trendelenburg.

C. DISADVANTAGES

1. Location depends on feeling femoral artery pulse or blindly estimating location of femoral artery.

2. Complication rate is higher than for peripheral veins (e.g., vein infection in the legs).

D. TECHNIQUE FOR CANNULATION

1. *Locate the artery.* The femoral artery is located by palpation with two fingers or by blind estimation of the midpoint between the symphysis pubis and the anterior iliac spine. The vein is immediately medial to the artery (Figure 4.51).

2. *Prep the skin.* The skin is prepped with iodine and then alcohol, although sterility during a Code Blue effort is hard to maintain.

3. *Insert the needle.* The catheter-over-needle set attached to a 10-ml syringe is directed at a 60-degree angle between the syringe and the long axis of the thigh (Figure

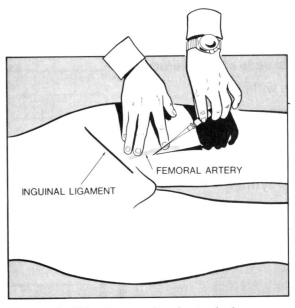

Figure 4–52   Femoral vein technique.

4.52). The needle enters the skin with the bevel facing the head. The needle is directed in until it stops against firm tissue. In this way the vein is pierced. Then with steady back pressure of syringe aspiration the catheter and needle are slowly withdrawn until blood freely enters the syringe.

4. *Lower the needle.* Next, the needle and catheter are lowered until they lie along the thigh parallel to the frontal plane. If blood still returns upon reaspiration of the syringe, the catheter is advanced up the vein.

5. *Secure.* The syringe and needle are withdrawn. Then the syringe is reattached to the catheter to once more confirm free blood flow. Blood samples are taken at this time if needed. The IV is now connected and a free flow of fluid is observed. The IV is secured similarly to the method in the peripheral venipuncture section.

E. LAB PRACTICE. The following Femoral Vein Venipuncture Procedure Guide is provided to aid the student in lab practice of this technique. Unless a suitable manikin is available, much of the lab practice will involve discussion of technique. This would be a good procedure for the cadaver setting. Paired students take turns being rescuer and evaluator.

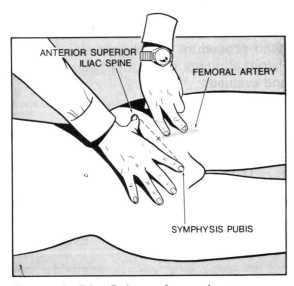

Figure 4–51   Palpate femoral artery.

FEMORAL VEIN VENIPUNCTURE PROCEDURE GUIDE

Rescuer's Name _____ Date _____ Evaluator _____

Directions for Evaluator: Place a check beside each item whenever an exam step is omitted, or performed improperly, or presented improperly.

Step	Method	Evaluation
1. Locate the artery	a. Palpate artery.	_____
	b. Indicate vein is medial.	_____
2. Prep the skin	a. Prep skin with iodine.	_____
	b. Finish prep with alcohol.	_____
3. Insert the needle	a. Direct catheter-over-needle at a 60-degree angle.	_____
	b. Keep bevel toward head.	_____
	c. Proceed until firm tissue is encountered.	_____
	d. Aspirate as needle is withdrawn.	_____
4. Lower the needle	a. Lower syringe and needle.	_____
	b. Retest blood return.	_____
	c. Advance catheter up vein.	_____
5. Secure	a. Withdraw needle and syringe.	_____
	b. Attach syringe to catheter.	_____
	c. Reaspirate.	_____
	d. Take blood samples.	_____
	e. Connect IV line.	_____
	f. Observe free IV fluid flow.	_____
	g. Secure IV as before.	_____

Subclavian Vein

A. ANATOMY. The subclavian vein is a branch of the brachiocephalic vein (innominate; Figure 4.53). On the left side the thoracic duct terminates into the venous system at this juncture, thus making the right side the usual preference for the first attempt.

The subclavian vein runs anterior to the anterior scalene muscle, whereas the subclavian artery lies posterior to the muscle. This makes the vein accessible to needles passed under the clavicle.

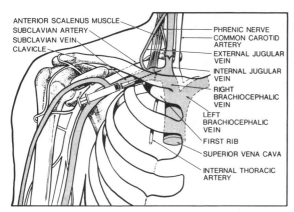

Figure 4-53 Anatomy of subclavian vein.

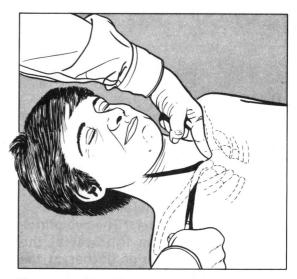

Figure 4-54 Subclavian vein technique.

Medial to the scalene muscle are such structures as the apical pleura, phrenic nerve, internal thoracic artery, and others. These structures must be avoided; emphasize the need for the paramedic to stay just beneath the clavicle.

B. ADVANTAGES.
1. Does not require vein visualization or artery palpation

2. Rapid access to central circulation

C. DISADVANTAGES.
1. Must stop CPR

2. Pneumothorax common

D. TECHNIQUE FOR CANNULATION. Although the subclavian vein can be approached from above the clavicle, the most common approach is from below (Figure 4.54).

1. *Locate landmarks.* The first landmark is the juncture of the medial third and middle third of the clavicle. Recently, a special tubercle has been described at this juncture, which can be palpated in many people. This location marks the place at which the needle is directed below the clavicle. Skin entrance is 1 cm inferior and 1 cm lateral to this location so that the needle can skate just below the clavicle.

The second landmark is the suprasternal notch, which is often determined and marked with a finger throughout the procedure. This marks the direction toward which the needle is advanced.

2. *Prep the skin.* The skin is prepped with iodine followed with alcohol. A large margin is prepped since it is easy to touch unprepped skin in this area, as the needle is parallel to the skin most of the time. Trendelenburg or antishock trousers are used to fill the veins.

3. *Insert the needle.* The needle enters the skin at the location mentioned above. Every effort is made to lower the shoulder so that the needle can indeed be parallel to the skin of the chest wall. The needle is directed toward the suprasternal notch as the attached syringe is aspirated. After there is blood return the needle and catheter are advanced 3 mm to make sure that the catheter is in the vein as well.

4. *Advance the catheter.* The catheter is now advanced into the subclavian vein.

5. *Secure.* The syringe and needle are withdrawn. Then the syringe is reattached to the catheter and once more free flow of blood is confirmed. Blood samples are taken at this time. If there is not free flow of blood, the catheter is removed. At no time is the hub of the catheter left exposed to the air as air embolism can easily occur.

The IV is now connected and free flow of fluid is observed. The IV is secured similarly to the method in the peripheral venipuncture section. Secure to chest, not arm, to prevent separation of IV tubing from catheter hub.

E. LAB PRACTICE. The following Subclavian Vein Venipuncture Procedure Guide is provided to aid the student in lab practice of this technique. This would be a good procedure for the cadaver setting. Paired students take turns being rescuer and evaluator. In the absence of suitable manikins, much of the lab practice will involve discussion of the technique. At the very least the anatomy should be drawn on plastic wrap placed over a fellow student's upper torso.

Internal Jugular Vein (Posterior Approach)

A. ANATOMY. The internal jugular vein is a branch of the brachiocephalic vein (innominate; Figures 4.55 and 4.56). Once again the proximity of the thoracic duct termination on the left encourages most rescuers to try the right side first.

The internal jugular vein lies lateral and slightly anterior to the carotid artery in the

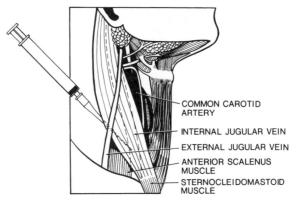

Figure 4–56   Internal jugular technique.

inferior part of the neck, where it is cannulated. The vein is covered in its course by the sternocleidomastoid muscle.

As the anterior approach is difficult due to the presence of the jaw and the inferior approach is more risky to deep structures, most rescuers prefer the posterior approach behind the sternocleidomastoid.

B. ADVANTAGES.
1. No need to visualize vein

2. Large vein

3. Rapid access to central circulation

C. DISADVANTAGES.
1. Risk of bleeding, nerve damage, or tracheal damage

2. Head must be turned and patient in Trendelenburg

3. Hard to secure

D. TECHNIQUE FOR CANNULATION.

1. *Locate Landmarks.* The two principal landmarks are as follows: (a) the juncture of the posterior border of the sternocleidomastoid muscle and the external jugular vein, and (b) the suprasternal notch. The skin entrance site is just superior to the vein–muscle junction.

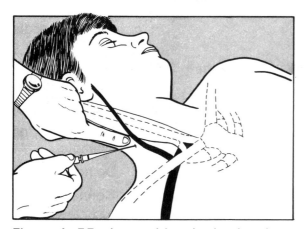

Figure 4–55   Internal jugular landmarks.

SUBCLAVIAN VEIN VENIPUNCTURE PROCEDURE GUIDE

Rescuer's Name _____ Date _____ Evaluator _____

Directions for Evaluator: Place a check beside each item whenever an exam step is omitted, or performed improperly, or presented improperly.

Step	Method	Evaluation
1. Locate landmarks	a. Identify junction of middle third and medial third of clavicle.	_____
	b. Identify skin entrance point.	_____
	c. Locate suprasternal notch.	_____
2. Prep the skin	a. Prep the skin with iodine.	_____
	b. Finish the prep with alcohol.	_____
	c. Put patient in Trendelenburg position or inflate antishock trousers to fill veins.	_____
3. Insert the needle	a. Insert the needle through skin.	_____
	b. Direct the needle under the clavicle toward the suprasternal notch.	_____
	c. Advance needle 3 mm past point of aspirated blood return.	_____
4. Advance the catheter	a. Advance the catheter into the subclavian vein.	_____
5. Secure	a. Withdraw the syringe and needle.	_____
	b. Reattach syringe and withdraw blood sample.	_____
	c. Do not expose open catheter hub to air.	_____
	d. Connect IV tubing.	_____
	e. Secure IV to chest, not arm.	_____

2. *Prep the Skin.* The skin is prepped with iodine followed with alcohol. Trendelenburg or antishock trousers are used to fill the veins.

3. *Insert the Needle.* The needle is inserted at the skin entrance site described above. The needle is passed just beneath the sternocleidomastoid muscle aiming toward the suprasternal notch. The vein is usually cannulated at about 6 cm inferior to the skin entrance site.

After there is blood return, the needle and catheter are advanced 3 mm more to make sure that the catheter is in the vein well.

4. *Advance the Catheter.* The catheter is now advanced over the needle into the internal jugular vein.

The syringe and needle are withdrawn. Then the syringe is reattached to the catheter and once more free flow of blood is confirmed. Blood samples are taken at this time. If there is not free flow of blood, the catheter is removed. At no time is the hub of the catheter left exposed to the air as air embolism can easily occur.

5. *Secure.* The IV line is now connected and free flow of fluid must be observed. The IV is secured similarly to the method in the peripheral venipuncture section. Be sure that the head can move and not dislodge the IV tubing.

E. LAB PRACTICE. The following Internal Jugular Vein Venipuncture Procedure Guide is provided to aid the student in lab practice of this technique. This would be a good procedure for the cadaver setting. Paired students take turns being rescuer and evaluator. In the absence of suitable manikins, much of the lab practice will involve discussion of the technique. At the very least the anatomy should be drawn on plastic wrap placed over a fellow student's upper torso.

SUMMARY*

The circulatory system involves three components: the heart, the blood vessels, and blood itself. This chapter has dealt primarily with methods of increasing effective blood volume. Antishock trousers transfer available blood from the legs and abdomen to the upper torso to improve perfusion of the brain and heart. A trauma IV adds a salt solution to replace loss of blood volume or fluid. In the situation of internal bleeding where basic skills of compression and elevation cannot be used, shock trousers and trauma IVs remain temporary measures to get a patient to the surgical skills needed to stop the bleeding.

*The primary reference for the central vein techniques was the excellent Chapter XII of the *Advanced Cardiac Life Support* text. This chapter, written by William Kaye, M.D., helped the senior author to improve his own technique on all three of the central vein skills discussed in this chapter of the *Paramedic Skills Manual*.

INTERNAL JUGULAR VEIN VENIPUNCTURE PROCEDURE GUIDE

Rescuer's Name _____ Date _____ Evaluator _____

Directions for Evaluator: Place a check beside each item whenever an exam step is omitted, or performed improperly, or presented improperly.

Step	Method	Evaluation
1. Locate landmarks	a. Identify the sternocleidomastoid muscle.	_____
	b. Identify the external jugular vein.	_____
	c. Identify the suprasternal notch.	_____
	d. Explain that the skin entrance site is just superior to the junction of No. 1 and No. 2.	_____
2. Prep the skin	a. Prep the skin with iodine.	_____
	b. Finish the prep with alcohol.	_____
	c. Put the patient in Trendelenburg position or inflate antishock trousers to fill veins.	_____
3. Insert the needle	a. Insert the needle through skin.	_____
	b. Pass the needle just below the sternocleidomastoid muscle.	_____
	c. Advance the needle 3 mm past the point of aspirated blood return.	_____
4. Advance the catheter	a. Advance the catheter into the internal jugular vein.	_____
5. Secure	a. Withdraw the syringe and needle.	_____
	b. Reattach syringe and withdraw blood sample.	_____
	c. Do not expose open catheter hub to the air.	_____
	d. Connect IV tubing.	_____
	e. Secure IV so that it will not come out if the head is turned.	_____

SKILL PROFICIENCY TESTING

Skill   Antishock Trousers (Figure 4.57)

Performance   Demonstrate how to put on, maintain, and remove antishock trousers.

Conditions   1.   Manikin* in shock from a ruptured tubal pregnancy.

2.   Base hospital has confirmed that antishock trousers should be applied.

3.   Antishock trousers available in manufacturer's case.

4.   Blood pressure cuff and stethoscope available near patient.

5.   Initial blood pressure is 80/40 and pulse 120 and weak.

6.   Rescuer positions self near patient's feet until told to begin.

Standard   1.   Rescuer follows Antishock Trousers Procedure Guide, omitting no more than three steps.   ☐

2.   Time limit: 3 minutes.   ☐

*Some physicians feel that it is not safe to pump up the trousers on a simulated patient.

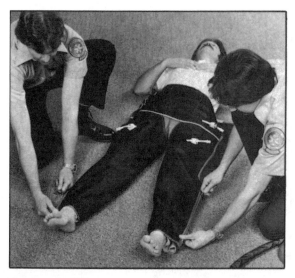

Figure 4–57

Student's Name _____ Date _____ Evaluator _____

Pass/Fail

SKILL PROFICIENCY TESTING

Skill   Peripheral Venipuncture (Figure 4.58)

Performance   Demonstrate how to prepare, insert, and troubleshoot a trauma IV.

Conditions
1. An assortment of IV equipment is available at least sufficient to start a trauma IV and a medical IV.
2. A patient, volunteer, or manikin's arm is available for IV insertion.
3. The evaluator explains that the base hospital just ordered a trauma IV. (The order has not yet been confirmed.)
4. Simulated radio or phone available for base hospital communication; evaluator simulates base hospital to give order for IV.
5. Evaluator also available to hold IV bag.

Standard
1. Rescuer starts IV according to the Detailed Peripheral Venipuncture Guide omitting no more than seven steps.   ☐

2. Time limit: Insertion   3 min   ☐

                    Securing   1 min   ☐

           Troubleshooting   1 min   ☐

Pass if follows Guide, starts IV, and meets time limits.

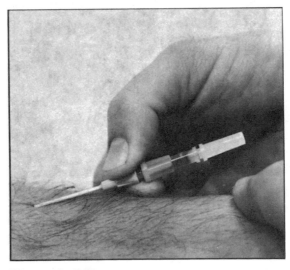

Figure 4-58

Student's Name _____ Date _____ Evaluator _____

Pass/Fail

SKILL PROFICIENCY TESTING

Skill   Femoral Vein Cannulation (Figure 4.59)

Performance   Demonstrate how to diagram and explain the cannulation of the femoral vein to obtain a central vein IV.

Conditions   1. Evaluator explains rescuer is to demonstrate anatomy without perforating skin.

2. Volunteer with towel over genitals.

3. Plastic wrap available over groin.

4. Magic markers—red and blue.

5. Rescuer is to draw the anatomy—red (artery) and blue (vein).

6. A 6-inch catheter-over-needle with a 10-cc syringe.

Standard   1. Rescuer follows Femoral Vein Procedure Guide, omitting no more than three steps.   ☐

2. Time limit: 2 minutes.   ☐

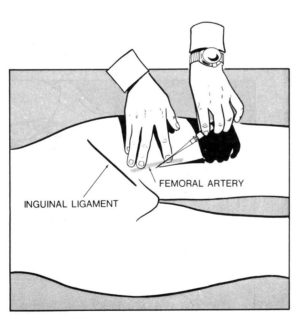

FEMORAL ARTERY

INGUINAL LIGAMENT

Figure 4–59

Student's Name _____ Date _____ Evaluator _____

Pass/Fail

SKILL PROFICIENCY TESTING

Skill Subclavian Vein Cannulation (Infraclavicular Approach; Figure 4.60)

Performance Demonstrate how to diagram and explain the cannulation of the left subclavian vein to obtain a central IV.

Conditions
1. Evaluator explains rescuer is to demonstrate anatomy without perforating skin.
2. Volunteer.
3. Plastic wrap placed over left clavicle.
4. Magic markers—brown, red, blue.
5. Rescuer is to draw anatomy and explain procedure.
6. A 6-inch catheter-over-needle with a 10-cc syringe for demonstration but not actual skin penetration.

Standard
1. Rescuer draws on Saran wrap to demonstrate anatomy: brown (muscle), red (artery), and blue (vein). ☐
2. Rescuer follows Subclavian Vein Procedure Guide, omitting no more than three steps. ☐
3. Time limit: 2 minutes. ☐

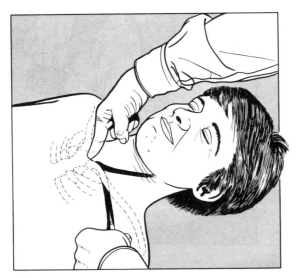

Figure 4–60

Student's Name _____ Date _____ Evaluator _____

Pass/Fail

SKILL PROFICIENCY TESTING

Skill   Internal Jugular Cannulation (Posterior Approach; Figure 4.61)

Performance   Demonstrate how to diagram and explain cannulation of the internal jugular vein in order to obtain a central vein IV.

Conditions
1. Evaluator explains rescuer is to demonstrate anatomy without perforating skin.
2. Volunteer with upper chest and neck bare.
3. Plastic wrap available over neck.
4. Magic markers—red, blue, and brown.
5. Rescuer to draw the anatomy: red (artery), blue (vein), and brown (muscle).
6. A 6-inch catheter-over-needle with a 10-cc syringe.

Standard
1. Rescuer follows Internal Jugular Vein Procedure Guide, omitting no more than three steps.   ☐
2. Time limit: 2 minutes.   ☐

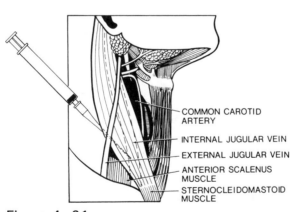

COMMON CAROTID ARTERY
INTERNAL JUGULAR VEIN
EXTERNAL JUGULAR VEIN
ANTERIOR SCALENUS MUSCLE
STERNOCLEIDOMASTOID MUSCLE

Figure 4–61

Student's Name _____ Date _____ Evaluator _____

Pass/Fail

5

Medication Administration

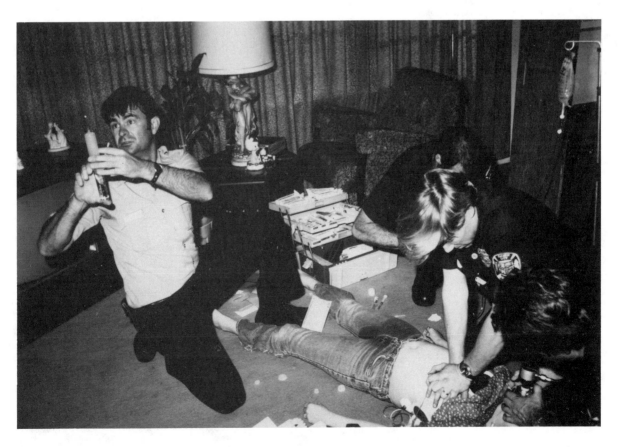

Skills Objectives

- **Subcutaneous Injection** — Demonstrate how to administer 0.3 cc of 1:1000 epinephrine (simulated) using an ampule and tuberculin syringe.

- **Intramuscular Injection** — Demonstrate how to inject 5 mg of morphine intramuscularly using a Tubex syringe.

- **Intravenous Preload Bolus Administration** — Demonstrate how to administer 100 mg of lidocaine by IV bolus using a preloaded syringe.

- **Intravenous Piggyback Drip** — Demonstrate how to administer 2 g of lidocaine in 500 cc of D_5W by IV piggyback drip.

- **Endotracheal Medication Administration** — Demonstrate how to administer appropriate drugs via ET tube.

- **Inhalation Analgesia** — Demonstrate how to administer nitrous oxide.

Outline

Medication Administration Skills Description

INTRODUCTION

The skills associated with giving correct medications are some of the most important skills in advanced life support. Errors in drug concentrations, misreading labels, giving medications through an IV that is not working, and so on, can all have life-threatening consequences. The paramedic must develop good habits to try to avoid such errors as much as possible. Errors, however, may be made and it is important to inform the base hospital immediately in this event.

Many of these errors can be minimized in a paramedic system by limiting the number of drugs carried and by using preloaded syringes as much as possible. Using morphine in the Tubex preload system avoids having two ampules—morphine and adrenalin—that look alike being side by side in the same drug box. Even IV solution choices should be limited so that errors are minimized; for example, carrying only 1000 cc of Ringer's lactate and 500 cc of dextrose 5% in water. The difference in the two sizes prevents errors. The best protection, however, is always to check medications and solutions prior to use.

SPECIAL CONSIDERATIONS

The following points should be remembered by paramedics responsible for administering drugs:

1. The drugs paramedics carry are among the most potent in medicine and should be treated with respect.

2. It is better to have no IV than to think that an IV is working when it is infiltrated.

3. Never give a cloudy medication intravenously.

4. Confirm all medication orders before administration and again after administration, the second time noting any effects.

5. Medications given during cardiac arrest will not get to the heart muscle unless they are perfused by CPR.

6. Once a needle has entered a patient it presents the possible risk of having picked up hepatitis viruses and recapping or using prepackaged disposable units must be a critical skill.

7. Prior to administration, recheck type of drug, dose, route, and expiration date.

8. Paramedics need to have a close working relationship with the hospital pharmacist since their drugs are exposed to many variables, such as heat and cold, which make usual expiration dates unreliable.

Addicting Drugs

Paramedics invariably carry drugs such as morphine and diazepam (Valium) which are potentially addicting. This makes the possibility of theft very high. Every community will have to devise its own method of records to satisfy federal, state, and local regulations. Paramedics must realize that this is important and for their own protection.

OVERVIEW OF SEQUENCES

The attempt in this chapter is to devise a common pattern for the various routes of drug administration. The pattern chosen is as follows:

Confirm the Order

Each order has to be confirmed before it can be followed. If an order seems out of place, it should be questioned once. If an order is likely to do harm, it must not be followed. Even when protocol sequences are worked out, each separate drug must be mentioned by name, dose, and route.

Prepare the Medication

Most patients are reassured if they understand that they are getting a medication to help them feel better. Also, just before giving a medication, it is important to recheck allergies. Other steps are designed around giving the medication by the proper route, maintaining sterility, and handling the needle safely after use.

Administer the Medication

The medication is delivered carefully. If given into an IV portal, the drip must be turned up briefly to get the medication into the vein circulation.

Confirm Medication Administration

After a medication is given, its administration should be confirmed. Often there is no immediate effect, but when there is, it should be noted.

MEDICATION ROUTES

Medication routes are generally chosen related to speed of action. For most situations

in critical care, the intravenous route is preferred because it is the most dependable. Giving adrenalin subcutaneously for asthma and morphine intramuscularly for extremity fracture without shock are unusual exceptions. Some of the time elements are compared in Tables 5.1 and 5.2.

Subcutaneous Injection

The subcutaneous route is rarely used in emergency situations, especially shock, because of uneven absorption and therefore

Table 5.1. ROUTE VERSUS TIME.

Route	Example	Time of Effect	Typical Clinical Situation
Oral	Ipecac	20 minutes	Child swallows iron pills
Subcutaneous	Epinephrine	15 minutes	Young adult with asthma
Intramuscular	Morphone	10 minutes	Young adult with broken arm
Intravenous push	Lidocaine	1 minute	Heart patient with irritability of ventricle
Intravenous drip	Isoproferenal	1 minute	Heart patient with symptoms and conduction block
Sublingual injection	Epinephrine	3 minutes	Severe allergic reaction; no time to start IV
Endotracheal	Ephinephrine	2 minutes	Cardiac arrest; unable to get IV in
Intracardiac	Epinephrine	15 seconds	Cardiac arrest; unable to get IV or endotracheal tube in; ET tube not inserted
Inhalation	Nitrous oxide	3 minutes	Patient with limb fracture

Table 5.2. ROUTE VERSUS COMPLICATION POTENTIAL.

Route	Location	Advantages	Disadvantages
Oral	Per mouth	No needles	Slow effect
Subcutaneous	Deltoid subcut	Faster than oral	Unpredictable absorption in shock
Intramuscular	Deltoid muscle	Faster than subcutaneous	Still unpredictable absorption in shock; also interferes with some cardiac muscle tests
Intravenous	Any IV	Very fast and predictable	Side effects may be very severe
Endotracheal	Trachea	No need for IV	Not all medications are cleared for this site

unpredictability. One of the few exceptions to this is epinephrine for asthma. Epinephrine is so strong that it can have a dramatic effect even subcutaneously.

JUDGMENT

Indications

In asthma, epinephrine is appropriately given subcutaneously, as it does not require an IV.

Contraindications

The skin should not be punctured if it is injured (e.g., a burn) or infected; a patient in shock should not have a subcutaneous medication, due to very slow absorption.

Precautions

As always, check allergy to medications, use aseptic technique, and use the standard safety steps of repeating doses, reading labels, and so on. Pick areas of the body such as the deltoid region of the upper arm where there are no major veins, arteries, or nerves near the skin. Consider aspirating syringe before injecting medication.

Complications

Infection, tissue irritation, and inadvertent IV administration are possible complications of subcutaneous injection.

EQUIPMENT

The equipment needed for this skill includes an ampule of epinephrine in 1:1000 concentration, a 1-cc tuberculin syringe with No. 25 needle, 2 × 2 gauze, an alcohol sponge, and a volunteer's arm. (During practice sterile water or saline should be substituted for epinephrine.)

SKILL SEQUENCE

The skill sequence should be separated into four sequential phases: confirming the order, preparing the medication, administering the medication, and confirming medication administration.

Confirm the Order

The rescuer is responsible to refuse any order that is grossly inconsistent with his or her training or may likely cause severe harm to the patient. This should be a rare event and does not suggest that the paramedic's judgment generally exceeds the physician's. If the order seems appropriate or at least unlikely to do harm, it should be confirmed (Figure 5.1) by repeating the medication, dosage, and route. For example,

> John Muir Base this is Pomeroy 22 confirming the order for 0.3 mg of epinephrine to be given subcutaneously.

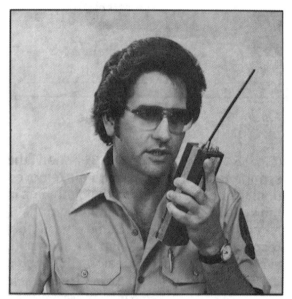

Figure 5–1   Confirming the order.

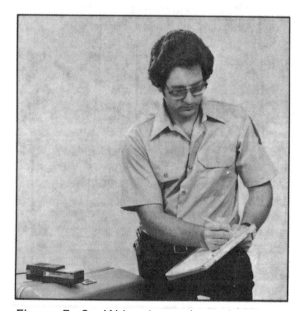

Figure 5–2   Write down the order.

The order is then written down, including the time (Figure 5.2).

Prepare the Medication

Proper preparation of a medication begins with obtaining a syringe, selecting the medication, checking the name, reading the name, and examining for cloudiness and expiration date (Figures 5.3 to 5.5). Since paramedic drug boxes are exposed to high and low temperatures, medications may deteriorate prior to the expiration date. A pharmacy committee must work with the paramedics to evaluate potential problems.

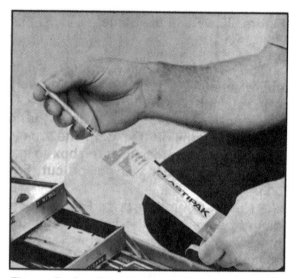

Figure 5–3   Obtain the syringe and needle.

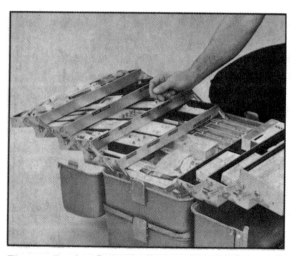

Figure 5–4   Select the medication.

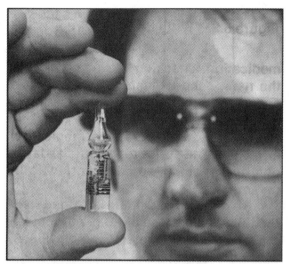

Figure 5–5   Read the name.

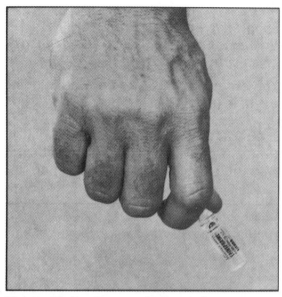

Figure 5–7   Rotate the ampule.

Next, the tip of the ampule is tapped to get fluid down to the bottom (Figure 5.6). Alternatively, the ampule may be rotated rapidly (Figure 5.7). This is particularly important if an entire ampule is to be given. To avoid being cut, the paramedic should use 2 × 2 gauze or an alcohol sponge to grasp the tip while breaking it off (Figure 5.8). The broken tip must be returned to the drug box so that the patient and rescuer will not be cut (Figure 5.9).

Now the ampule is tipped and the needle introduced into the liquid. Many ampules may be held upside down without spilling. The paramedic should try not to touch the needle to the edge of the ampule. The fluid is drawn up to more than the amount desired to allow for the air volume (Figure 5.10 to 5.13). Then the syringe is inverted and extra air removed until the correct volume of fluid

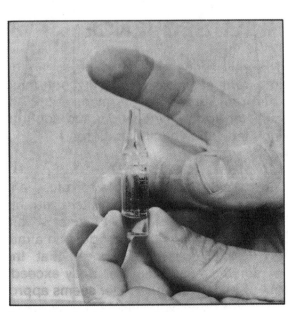

Figure 5–6   Tap the tip.

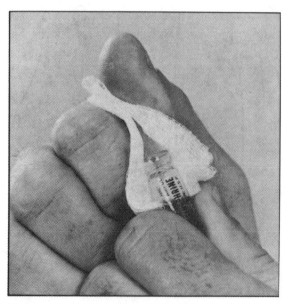

Figure 5–8   Break off the tip.

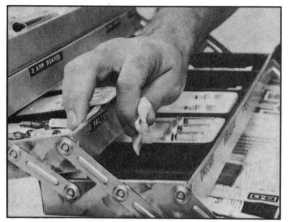

Figure 5-9 Return broken glass.

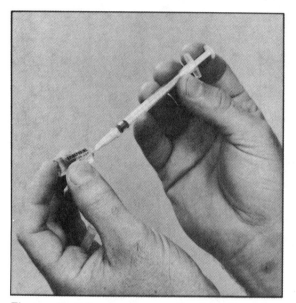

Figure 5-10 Insert needle downward.

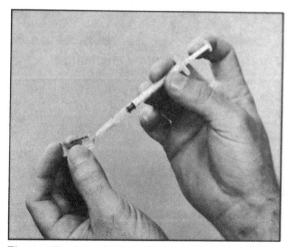

Figure 5-11 Withdraw medication.

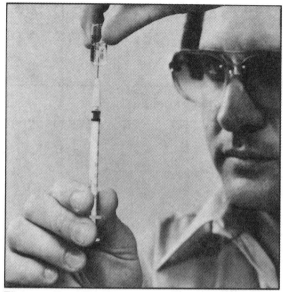

Figure 5-12 Insert needle in inverted ampule.

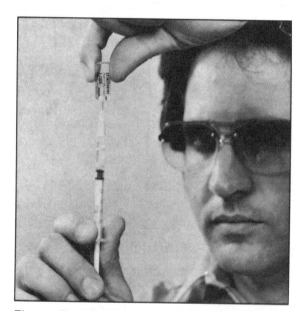

Figure 5-13 Withdraw medication.

remains in the syringe (Figure 5.14). Then the syringe is recapped (Figure 5.15). (Some instructors recommend that 0.2 cc of air be left in a syringe to avoid leaving medication along the needle track upon withdrawal.) Now the syringe is recapped. The opened ampule is returned to the drug box.

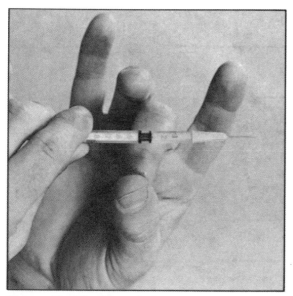

Figure 5-14 Expel air.

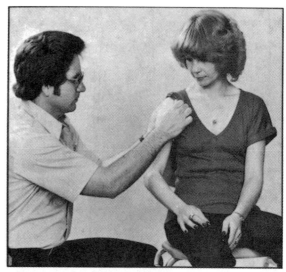

Figure 5-16 Expose deltoid.

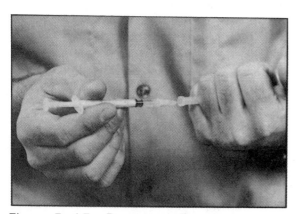

Figure 5-15 Recap needle.

Administer the Medication

The patient should be informed and reassured about the medication being given. Allergies should be rechecked even though done during patient exam. The shoulder is prepared by using an alcohol sponge in a concentric spiral starting at the proposed injection site (Figures 5.16 and 5.17).

The syringe cap is removed but kept in the paramedic's fingers for later recapping. The needle is inserted at 45 degrees, stopping after going through the dermis with the skin pulled away from the muscle (Figure

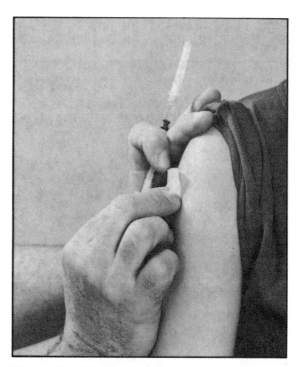

Figure 5-17 Prep deltoid.

5.18). The short TB syringe needle is usually inserted to the hub to prevent intradermal injection. The syringe is aspirated to make sure that there is no blood return (Figure 5.19). The medication is injected slowly (Figure 5.20). The needle should be

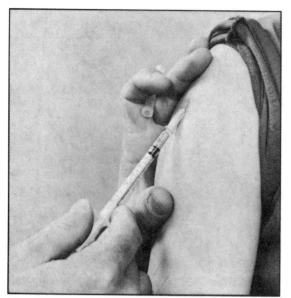

Figure 5–18   Insert needle.

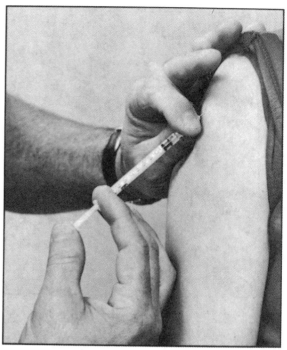

Figure 5–20   Inject medication.

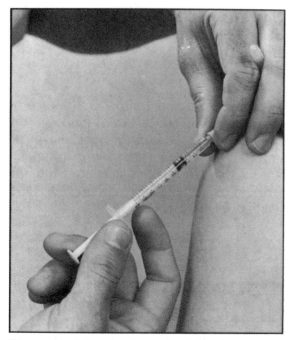

Figure 5–19   Aspirate for blood.

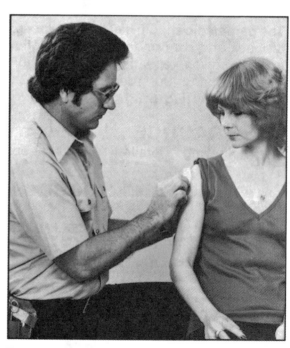

Figure 5–21   Apply pressure to site.

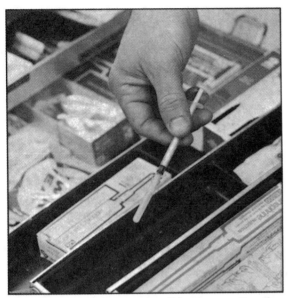

Figure 5-22   Return syringe to medication box.

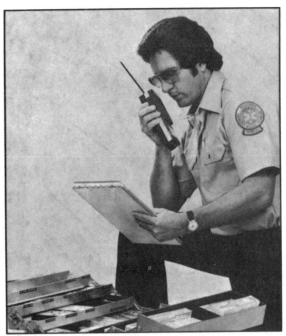

Figure 5-23   Confirm medication administration.

withdrawn quickly and the syringe recapped. (The most frequent cause of paramedics inadvertently sticking themselves with a used needle is careless or too rapid recapping.) Direct pressure is applied over the site of injection (Figure 5.21).

The syringe should be returned to the drug box (Figure 5.22). The needle has now been exposed to the patient and may be a carrier of such diseases as hepatitis. It should be treated with respect.

Confirm Medication Administration

The paramedic should call the base hospital back and confirm that the medication has been given, repeating the medication, the dose, and the route (Figure 5.23). Note patient change, if any.

LAB PRACTICE

The following Detailed Subcutaneous Medication Administration Guide is provided as an aid to lab practice of this skill. Sterile tuberculin syringes as well as ampules of saline resembling adrenalin are needed for this lab session. Students work in pairs, taking turns as rescuer and evaluator using the Guide.

DETAILED SUBCUTANEOUS MEDICATION ADMINISTRATION GUIDE

Rescuer's Name _____ Date _____ Evaluator _____

Directions for Evaluator: Place a check beside each item whenever an exam step is omitted, performed improperly, or presented improperly.

Step	**Method**	**Evaluation**
1. Confirm the order	a. Rescuer determines if the order is consistent with training.	_____
	b. Rescuer confirms order repeating:	_____
	(1) Medication	_____
	(2) Dosage	_____
	(3) Route	_____
	c. Rescuer writes down the order and the time.	_____
2. Prepare the medication	a. Obtains syringe with needle.	_____
	b. Selects epinephrine ampule and checks name.	_____
	c. Checks for cloudiness and expiration date.	_____
	d. Taps tip or rotates to get medication to the bottom.	_____
	e. Breaks off tip with 2 × 2 gauze.	_____
	f. Returns broken glass to medication box.	_____
	g. Inserts needle sterily.	_____
	h. Withdraws medication.	_____
	i. Expels air, leaving 0.3 cc of medication.	_____
	j. Recaps needle.	_____
	k. Returns rest of ampule to medication box.	_____

DETAILED SUBCUTANEOUS MEDICATION ADMINISTRATION GUIDE (Continued)

Rescuer's Name _____ Date _____ Evaluator _____

Step	Method	Evaluation
3. Administer the medication	a. Exposes the deltoid.	_____
	b. Reassures patient and rechecks allergies.	_____
	c. Preps the deltoid in spiral fashion.	_____
	d. Inserts the needle at 45 degrees.	_____
	e. Aspirates for blood.	_____
	f. Injects medication.	_____
	g. Applies pressure to the site.	_____
	h. Recaps syringe.	_____
	i. Returns syringe to medication box.	_____
4. Confirm medication administration	Confirms to simulated base hospital that medication has been given indicating:	
	a. Medication	_____
	b. Route	_____
	c. Dosage	_____
	d. Patient response	_____

Intramuscular Injection

An injection into a muscle is called an intramuscular (IM) injection. The three most common sites for such injections include the shoulder muscle (deltoid), the largest muscle of the buttocks (gluteous maximus), and the lateral thigh muscle (vastus lateralis). The most common site in the field would be the deltoid (Figure 5.24).

Few medications are given intramuscularly in the field. In heart attacks, lab

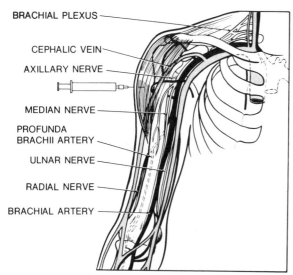

BRACHIAL PLEXUS

CEPHALIC VEIN

AXILLARY NERVE

MEDIAN NERVE

PROFUNDA
BRACHII ARTERY

ULNAR NERVE

RADIAL NERVE

BRACHIAL ARTERY

Figure 5-24   Anatomy of deltoid.

studies are altered by intramuscular injections. Also, in the trauma situation, intramuscular injections are discouraged because the patient may suddenly go into shock, making absorption very unpredictable. Therefore, intramuscular injections are not commonly given.

One of the few exceptions might be intramuscular morphine for the patient who has had a lower leg fracture with a good deal of pain. Morphine will not be discussed in this manual but rather the technique of intramuscular injections. Benadryl might also be given intramuscularly in moderate allergic reactions with itching but no hypotension.

JUDGMENT

Indications

Intramuscular injections are generally reserved for those situations in which the patient is not presumed to have a cardiac problem and the patient is not in shock. An example would be the administration of pain medication to the patient with a simple limb problem such as a fractured tibia or fractured wrist.

Contraindications

As mentioned previously, patients in shock should get IV medications only. Patients with small muscle mass may not have an appropriate site.

Precautions

Such structures as nerves, veins, and arteries should be avoided. The deltoid and lateral thigh are safe areas in this respect as compared to the buttocks. Some medications are very irritating to the muscles and are not commonly used in the prehospital setting.

Complications

The complications are the same as with those of subcutaneous injections (i.e., infection, tissue irritation, and inadvertent IV administration). Because the intramuscular injection is deeper in the body, the risk of such problems is greater.

EQUIPMENT

The equipment demonstrated in this step is the preloaded cartridge–syringe system. Although morphine also comes in ampules, such equipment was demonstrated in the section on subcutaneous injection. The preloaded Tubex equipment packaged by the Wyeth Drug Company involves a package of five loaded morphine cartridge needle units which they refer to as Tamp-r-tel. It is an example of a cartridge needle system.

With the Tubex system comes a Tubex hypodermic syringe, which will also be described (Figure 5.25). If a normal needle and syringe were used, the needle should be at least a No. 22 needle.

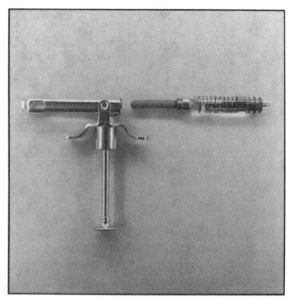

Figure 5–25 Tubex system.

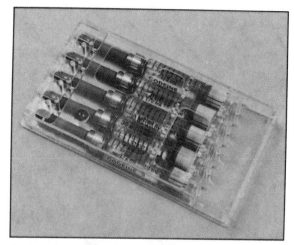

Figure 5–26 Tamp-R-Tel Systems

SKILL SEQUENCE

The skill sequence should be separated into the same phases as subcutaneous medication administration: confirm the order, prepare the medication, administer the medication, and confirm medication administration. Taught in this fashion the differences and similarities between the skills become clear.

Confirm the Order

The rescuer judges if the medication order is consistent with training guidelines. It should be questioned if the paramedic feels that it will do harm. If the medication seems appropriate, it is confirmed as to name, dosage, and route.

Prepare the Medication

The cartridge–needle unit is removed from a Tamp-r-tel pack (Figure 5.26). The paramedic reads the name of the drug and then

examines it for cloudiness and expiration date. Then the syringe is opened (Figure 5.27) and the cartridge–needle inserted (Figure 5.28). The cartridge has to be turned clockwise until it is threaded in (Figure 5.29).

Next the plunger is swung back into place and screwed onto the threaded shaft of the cartridge piston. The plunger is rotated further until the unit is fully engaged (Figure 5.30). Then the syringe is uncapped and the excess medication and air is expelled (Figure 5.31) The syringe is recapped until ready.

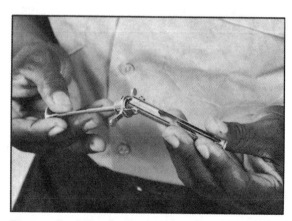

Figure 5–27 Swing handle downward.

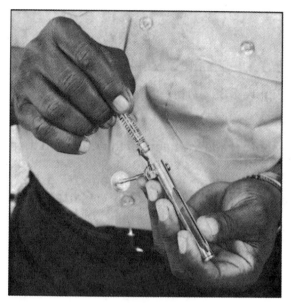

Figure 5-28   Insert cartridge.

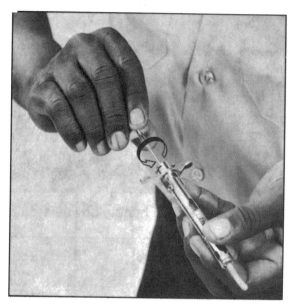

Figure 5-30   Thread plunger.

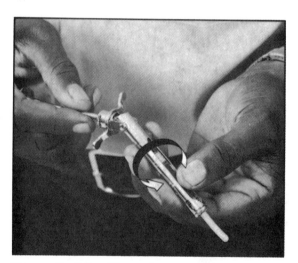

Figure 5-29   Thread cartridge.

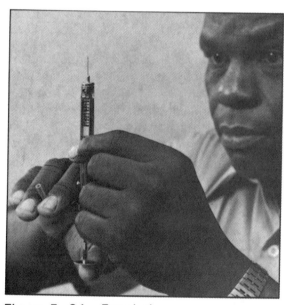

Figure 5-31   Expel air.

Administer the Medication

The paramedic explains to the patient what the medication is for and reassures the patient. Allergies are rechecked even though done during the patient exam. The deltoid area is prepared with the alcohol sponge moving in concentric circles (Figure 5.32). The syringe is uncapped and inserted at a *90-degree angle* into the muscle as the skin is pulled flat over the muscle (Figure 5.33).

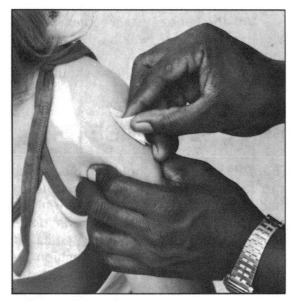

Figure 5-32   Prep skin.

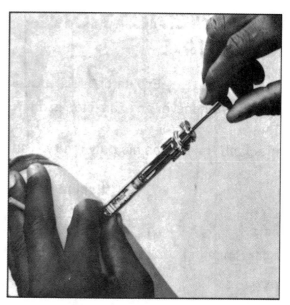

Figure 5-34   Check for blood return.

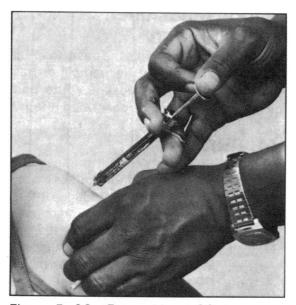

Figure 5-33   Enter skin at 90 degrees.

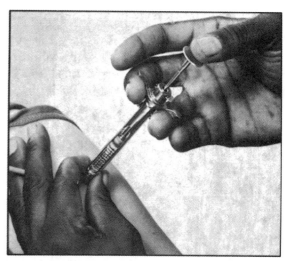

Figure 5-35   Inject medication.

The syringe is aspirated to make sure that there is no blood return. If there is blood return, the needle and syringe should be withdrawn and a new syringe and needle as well as a new site chosen for administra-tion of the medication (Figure 5.34). The medication is injected slowly (Figure 5.35). Once completed, the syringe is withdrawn quickly and needle recapped (Figure 5.36). This needle has been exposed to the patient

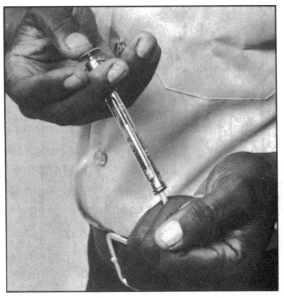

Figure 5-36   Withdraw and recap needle.

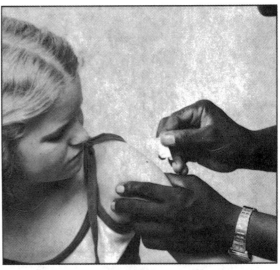

Figure 5-37   Massage injection site.

and must not stick the rescuer. Direct pressure is applied over the site of injection (Figure 5.37). The recapped syringe is returned to the drug box. If narcotics are used, the administered and discarded medication must be accounted for. Each EMS system will develop forms for such records.

Confirm Medication Administration

The paramedic then calls the base hospital back and indicates that the medication has been given. The name, dosage, route, and any effects should all be described briefly.

LAB PRACTICE

The following Detailed Intramuscular Medication Administration Guide is provided as an aid to lab practice of this skill. Sterile syringes and saline resembling morphine ampules are needed for this lab session. Students work in pairs, taking turns as rescuer and evaluator using the Guide.

DETAILED INTRAMUSCULAR MEDICATION ADMINISTRATION GUIDE

Rescuer's Name _____ Date _____ Evaluator _____

Directions for Evaluator: Place a check beside each item whenever an exam step is omitted, performed improperly, or presented improperly.

Sample Patient Problem: A 25-year-old male with a limb fracture as his only injury. The hospital has ordered morphine 7.5 mg IM.

Step	Method	Evaluation
1. Confirm the order	a. Rescuer determines if the order is consistent with training.	_____
	b. Rescuer confirms order repeating:	_____
	(1) Medication	_____
	(2) Dosage	_____
	(3) Route	_____
	c. Rescuer writes down the order and the time.	_____
2. Prepare the medication	a. Obtains Tubex syringe.	_____
	b. Selects Tamp-r-tel morphine package.	_____
	c. Opens package and removes one cartridge–needle.	_____
	d. Checks name.	_____
	e. Checks for cloudiness and expiration date.	_____
	f. Swings handle section downward.	_____
	g. Inserts cartridge.	_____
	h. Threads cartridge.	_____
	i. Threads plunger.	_____
	j. Uncaps and expels air.	_____
	k. Recaps.	_____

DETAILED INTRAMUSCULAR MEDICATION ADMINISTRATION GUIDE (Continued)

Rescuer's Name _____ Date _____ Evaluator _____

Step	Method	Evaluation
3. Administer the medication	a. Exposes deltoid.	_____
	b. Reassures the patient and rechecks allergies.	_____
	c. Preps deltoid in spiral fashion.	_____
	d. Inserts the needle at 90 degrees.	_____
	e. Aspirates for blood return.	_____
	f. Injects medication.	_____
	g. Withdraws and recaps needle.	_____
	h. Massages injection site.	_____
	i. Returns syringe to medication box.	_____
4. Confirm medication administration	a. Confirms to simulated base hospital that medication has been given indicating:	_____
	(1) Medication	_____
	(2) Route	_____
	(3) Dosage	_____
	(4) Patient response	_____

Intravenous Preload Bolus Administration

Over the last decade a number of medications have been prepared in preloaded syringes, eliminating the problem of drawing up medications and discarding small pieces of glass. Most cardiac medications are in a preloaded form, as is 50% dextrose and other noncardiac drugs. It would be convenient if all prehospital medications were preloaded, but it takes some time for the Food and Drug Administration to approve a change to preload form of any particular medication. The IV preload medication discussed in this section will be lidocaine; its particular properties, however, are not discussed in this book.

JUDGMENT
Indications

Preloaded medications are generally intravenous and are used when a very quick result is required. Lidocaine, for example, is used to decrease cardiac irritation. Once this irritability is discovered, the medication must be given very rapidly. The speed of action of preload medication is the same as all medication given intravenously—often 30 seconds to several minutes. More time is saved in the preparation of the medication.

Contraindications

The paramedic must be assured that the IV into which the medication is being added is working well or else the medication may go subcutaneously rather than IV. Many of these preload medications are very strong and can cause skin damage if this mistake occurs. An IV bolus is contraindicated where the patency of the IV is unclear.

Precautions

Since the preload medications look alike, special attention must be given to reading the label carefully. Special attention should be given to reviewing allergies as well.

Complications

Complications include giving the medication subcutaneously or dislodging the IV by pushing too hard. Actually, although this technique is also called pushing a medication in, the general rule is to administer the medication over 15 to 30 seconds.

EQUIPMENT

Preloaded syringes usually come in a box or plastic wrap containing two components side by side: one is the ampule filled with the medication and the second is the syringe barrel into which it is engaged and then injected (Figure 5.38). One or more companies

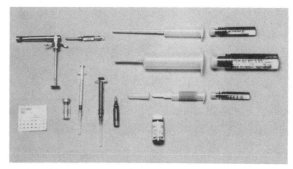

Figure 5-38   Preload kit vs. others.

market the syringe in a long container ready to engage. Many of the preload syringes have 3½-inch needles for intracardiac injection, although the Heart Association is trying to discourage this route. These long needles may also be broken off easily and the medication can be injected directly into the IV tubing. The medication should be used relatively quickly after opening the package, as the possibility of contamination increases with time.

SKILL SEQUENCE
Confirm the Order

The rescuer is responsible to refuse any order that is grossly inconsistent with his training or likely to cause severe harm to the patient. This should be a rare event and does not suggest that the paramedic's judgment generally exceeds the physician's. If the order seems appropriate or at least unlikely to do harm, it should be confirmed by repeating the medication, dosage, and route.

Prepare the Medication

The correct preload syringe is selected. (Figure 5.39) The name is read from the package and again once removed from the package (Figures 5.40 to 5.42) The syringe is checked for cloudiness and expiration date. The paramedic flips off the protective caps and engages the syringe (Figures 5.43 and 5.44). The paramedic removes the protective needle cap, expels air out of the syringe, and recaps the needle (Figures 5.45 to 5.47).

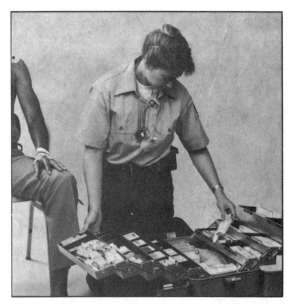

Figure 5-39   Select preload medication.

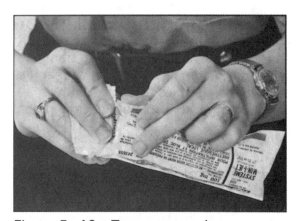

Figure 5-40   Tear open package.

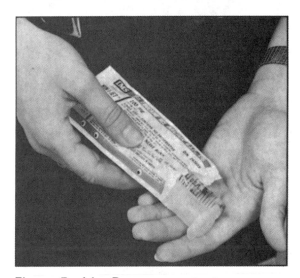

Figure 5-41   Remove contents.

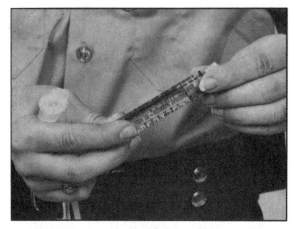

Figure 5-42   Read label.

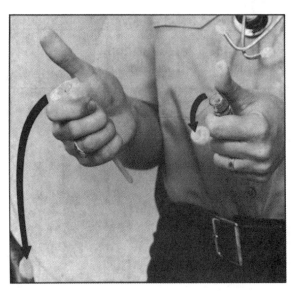

Figure 5-43   Flip off caps.

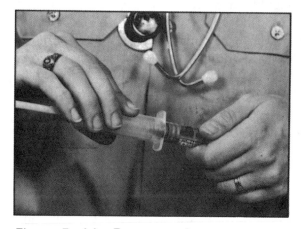

Figure 5-44   Engage syringe.

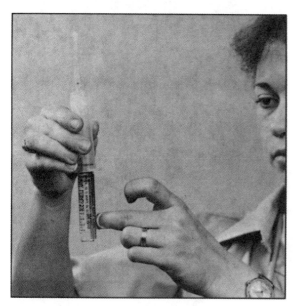

Figure 5–45   Tap air to top.

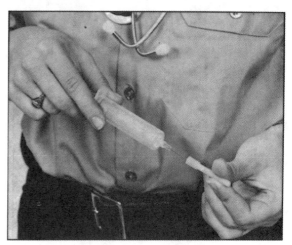

Figure 5–47   Recap needle.

Administer the Medication

The medication is explained to the patient and allergies rechecked. The paramedic selects an IV administration portal near the patient and cleanses the portal with an alcohol sponge (Figure 5.48). Rescuer notes that the main IV is running well. The syringe is injected into the portal (Figures 5.49 and 5.50), the tubing pinched off above this spot, and the medication is administered over 15 to 30 seconds while cloudiness is watched for in the tubing (Figure 5.51). The syringe is removed and recapped as the

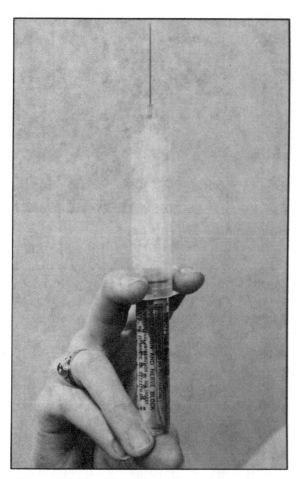

Figure 5–46   Expel air.

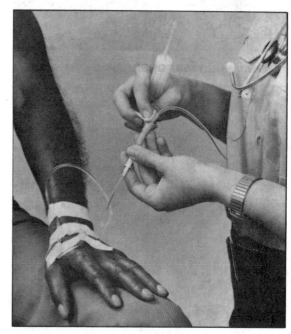

Figure 5–48   Prep portal.

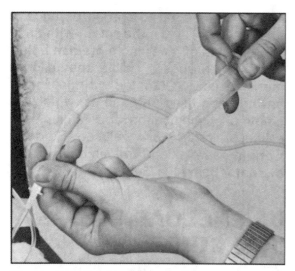

Figure 5-49   Uncap needle.

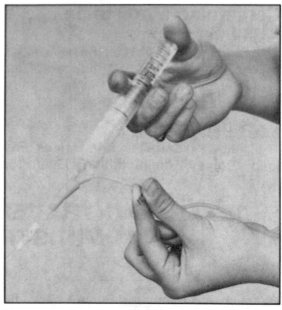

Figure 5-51   Pinch tubing and inject.

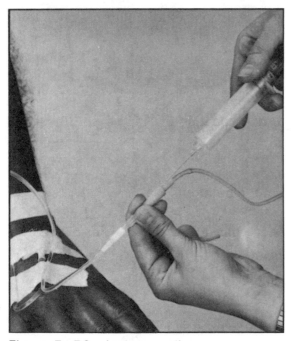

Figure 5-50   Insert needle.

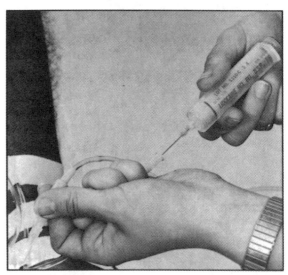

Figure 5-52   Recap needle and return to medication box.

tubing is released. The drip rate is speeded up briefly to flush all the medication in, and then turned back to 1 drip per second. The syringe is returned to the drug box (Figure 5.52.)

Confirm Medication Administration

The paramedic should call the base hospital back and confirm that the medication has been given, repeating the medication, the dose, and the route. Note the effect, if any.

LAB PRACTICE

The following Detailed Intravenous Preload Bolus Administration Guide is provided as an aid to lab practice of this skill. The lab can be set up with an IV arm capable of receiving a preload bolus. For safety purposes, saline should once more be used. Outdated syringes never having been used on patients, which are emptied of medication and refilled with saline or water, work well too. Students work in pairs, taking turns as rescuer and evaluator using the Guide.

DETAILED INTRAVENOUS PRELOAD BOLUS ADMINISTRATION GUIDE

Rescuer's Name _____ Date _____ Evaluator _____

Directions for Evaluator: Place a check beside each item whenever an exam step is omitted, performed improperly, or presented improperly.

Sample Patient Problem: A 60-year-old male with chest pain and multifocal premature ventricular beats. The hospital has ordered lidocaine 100 mg IV push.

Step	Method	Evaluation
1. Confirm the order	a. Rescuer determines if the order is consistent with training.	_____
	b. Rescuer confirms order repeating:	_____
	(1) Medication	_____
	(2) Dosage	_____
	(3) Route	_____
	c. Rescuer writes down the order and the time.	_____
2. Prepare the medication	a. Obtains correct preload package.	_____
	b. Tears open the package.	_____
	c. Removes the contents.	_____
	d. Reads the label.	_____
	e. Checks for cloudiness and expiration date.	_____
	f. Flips off the caps.	_____
	g. Engages the syringe.	_____
	h. Taps air to the top.	_____
	i. Uncaps and expels air.	_____
	j. Recaps preload.	_____

DETAILED INTRAVENOUS PRELOAD BOLUS ADMINISTRATION GUIDE (Continued)

Rescuer's Name _____ Date _____ Evaluator _____

Step	Method	Evaluation
3. Administer the medication	a. Identifies administration portal closest to the patient.	_____
	b. Preps the portal.	_____
	c. Uncaps the preload syringe, holding the cap off the ground to keep it sterile.	_____
	d. Inserts needle.	_____
	e. Pinches tubing above and slowly injects.	_____
	f. Recaps needle and returns preload to medication box.	_____
	g. Flushes tubing and then resets drip.	_____
4. Confirm medication administration	a. Confirms to simulated base hospital that medication has been given indicating:	
	(1) Medication	_____
	(2) Route	_____
	(3) Dosage	_____
	(4) Patient response	_____

Intravenous Piggyback Drip

Some medications are best given steadily over a long period. One example is the steady administration of a drug called dopamine for cardiogenic shock; the drug is given steadily with the dosage varied according to the blood pressure response. In this case the medication is added to an IV solution of dextrose and then piggybacked into a normal medical IV.

Another means of achieving the same goal is to inject a medication into the drip chamber of the IV tubing. Aminophyline is a drug sometimes used by paramedics in this way and is given over a 20-minute period.

This system of interposing a drip chamber (e.g., Volutrol or Metroset) allows additional control over inadvertent administration of a whole IV bag. Some systems use it as a standard for most drips other than lidocaine and dopamine. The author recommends that such a drip system be set up as a piggyback IV rather than the primary IV so that the piggyback line can be turned off without losing the IV, or use 50-cc IV solution bags for the piggyback line. The purpose of using the intravenous drip technique is that it allows the rescuer to maintain a constant drug level in the circulatory system.

JUDGMENT

Indications

Medication drips are indicated to either maintain a steady level of a certain medication or, because of a medication's potential toxicity, to give it over a period of time.

Contraindications

The usual contraindications deal with the properties of individual drugs rather than the route itself.

Precautions

The main precaution is to make sure that the main medical IV is functioning well. This medical IV should be turned off when the drip is going to avoid running the contents of one IV bag into another. If there is an adverse reaction to the piggybacked medication, it should be turned off and the main medical IV turned back on again.

Complications

As this IV is not being placed directly into the patient, complications relate primarily to the properties of the drug. A drip has to be monitored closely because changes in position often affect the drip rate.

EQUIPMENT

To prepare, for example, a lidocaine drip, the paramedic would need a microdrop drip chamber and a D_5W IV bag, a 2-g lidocaine preload syringe made to be injected into IV bottles or bags, a No. 22-needle and alcohol sponge to piggyback into another IV, some tape to hole it in place, and a method of labeling the IV bag.

SKILL SEQUENCE

As with other medication steps, the skill sequences can be divided into certain phases.

Confirm the Order

It is the rescuer's responsibility to refuse any order that is grossly inconsistent with his or her training or likely to cause severe harm to the patient. This should be a rare event and does not suggest that the paramedic's judgment generally exceeds the physician's. If the order seems appropriate or at least unlikely to do harm, it should be confirmed by repeating the medication, dosage, and route.

Prepare the Medication

Preparing the medication involves selection of the lidocaine 2-g syringe. This is opened, checked for name, date, expiration date, and cloudiness. Once the syringe of lidocaine is prepared, the administration portal of the D_5W IV bag should be cleansed with alcohol. Lidocaine is added to the D_5W IV bag. The syringe is removed, recapped, and safely placed back in the kit. The medication bag is labeled as to medication, amount added, and time of administration. A capped No. 22 needle is added to the end and the Iv tubing is flushed to be free of air bubbles. (Figures 5.53 to 5.58).

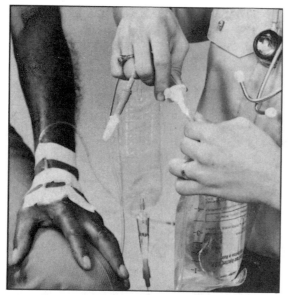

Figure 5–53 Obtain second IV bag and tubing.

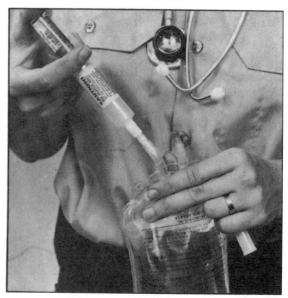

Figure 5–55 Inject medication into second bag.

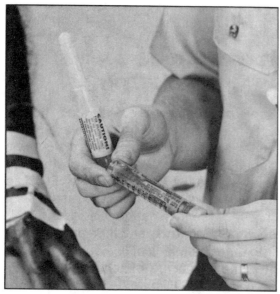

Figure 5–54 Read piggyback medication label.

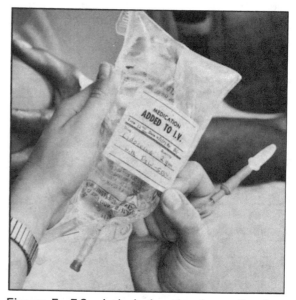

Figure 5–56 Label piggyback medication bag.

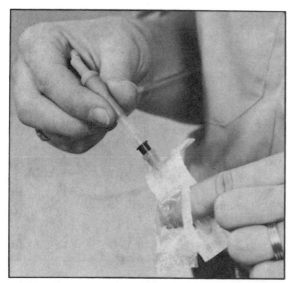

Figure 5–57 Connect needle to second IV line.

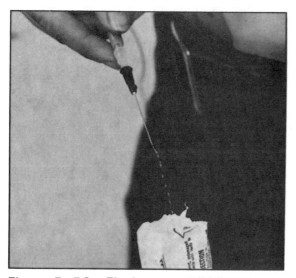

Figure 5–58 Flush second IV line.

Administer the Medication

The paramedic explains to the patient that an additional medication is being started. Allergies are rechecked. An IV administration portal of the main medical IV near the patient is selected. It is cleansed with alcohol, and the transfer needle inserted piggyback and taped in place (Figures 5.59 to 5.61). The main medical IV is closed off and

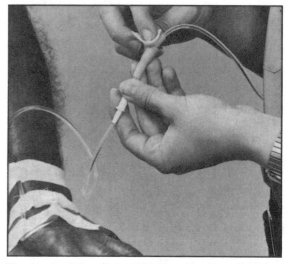

Figure 5–59 Prep IV portal in first IV line.

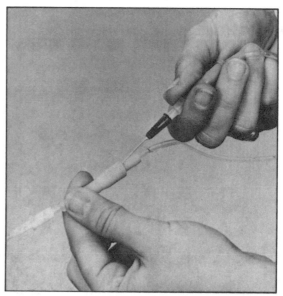

Figure 5–60 Insert piggyback needle into portal.

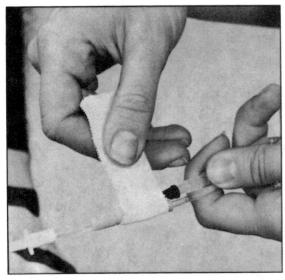

Figure 5-61   Tape piggyback needle in place.

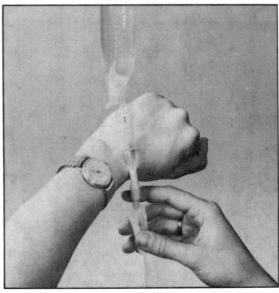

Figure 5-62   Set IV piggyback drip rate.

the piggyback drip is begun at the appropriate rate (Figure 5.62). All glass and used syringes are returned to the medication kit.

Confirm Medication Administration

The paramedic confirms to the base hospital that the medication has been given, indicating name, dosage, route, and response.

LAB PRACTICE

The following Detailed Intravenous Piggyback Medication Administration Guide is provided as an aid to lab practice of this skill. The lab can be set up with an IV arm with a medical IV already in place. The piggyback IV can then be set up by the student. Students work in pairs, taking turns as rescuer and evaluator using the Guide.

DETAILED INTRAVENOUS PIGGYBACK MEDICATION ADMINISTRATION GUIDE

Rescuer's Name _____ Date _____ Evaluator _____

Directions for Evaluator: Place a check beside each item whenever an exam step is omitted, performed improperly, or presented improperly.

Sample Patient Problem: A 68-year-old female who has developed chest pain with an episode of ventricular tachycardia. The burst of ventricular tachycardia was suppressed with a lidocaine push. The base hospital has now ordered a 4-mg/min lidocaine drip mixed 1 g of lidocaine in 500 cc of D_5W.

Step	Method	Evaluation
1. Confirm the order	a. Rescuer determines if the order is consistent with training.	_____
	b. Rescuer confirms order repeating:	_____
	(1) Medication	_____
	(2) Dosage	_____
	(3) Route	_____
	c. Rescuer writes down the order and the time.	_____
2. Prepare the medication	a. Obtains second IV bag and tubing.	_____
	b. Selects proper preload syringe.	_____
	c. Reads the label.	_____
	d. Checks for cloudiness and expiration date.	_____
	e. Opens IV bag IV tubing portal.	_____
	f. Injects preload drip medication.	_____
	g. Connects IV tubing to second bag.	_____
	h. Adds needle to second line.	_____
	i. Flushes line.	_____
3. Administer the medication	a. Identifies administration portal on first line closest to patient.	_____
	b. Preps portal.	_____
	c. Inserts piggyback needle into portal.	_____
	d. Tapes piggyback needle in place.	_____
	e. Turns off main medical IV.	_____
	f. Sets drip rate of piggyback IV.	_____

Endotracheal Medication Administration

Over the last decade a variety of medications have been given successfully through the endotracheal tube, including epinephrine, atropine, lidocaine, and naloxone. Direct absorption from the alveoli into the lung capillaries—the path of oxygen as well—has proven almost as effective as direct intravenous bolus of the same medication. *NAVEL* is the word that will remind you of the medications that can be administered: *n*aloxone, *a*tropine, *v*alium, *e*pinephrine, and *l*idocaine.

The steps used are not sufficiently different from the combination of endotracheal intubation and preload bolus administration to warrant a separate skill analysis. Thus a summary of skills is provided.

Technique

1. Oxygenate the patient.
2. Stop CPR.
3. Unhook the tube.
4. Instill the medication after exhalation.
5. Give positive pressure ventilation to dispense the medication.
6. Restart CPR.
7. Observe effects over the next 5 minutes.

Comment

The absorption of medication from this route is very rapid. It is appropriate to use if there is no IV or if the IV is not working well. Many of the medications used during cardiopulmonary arrest—such as lidocaine and epinephrine—can be used effectively this way. The small volumes of fluid do not seem to disturb oxygenation appreciably during the procedure.

CPR is stopped briefly during the procedure since vigorous chest compression can cause the medication to be pushed out of the endotracheal tube before it is dispersed down into the lung with positive pressure ventilation. In such a case the actual amount of medication delivered becomes very unclear.

Inhalation Analgesia (Nitrous Oxide)

Following effective utilization of nitrous oxide in prehospital care in countries such as England, its use in the United States has steadily increased. The principal difference is that two gas cannisters must be used in the United States due to variable temperature, whereas in England one cannister with oxygen and nitrous oxide mixed has worked well.

Safety in the use of nitrous oxide is enhanced by certain procedures:

1. Do not give it to intoxicated patients.
2. Avoid mixing it with other pain medications to avoid oversedation.
3. Have the patient self-administer the medication.
4. Vent ambulance to keep crews from becoming giddy.
5. Keep the medication locked up when not in use.

These and other precautions are discussed in more detail later.

JUDGMENT

Indications

Nitrous oxide is indicated for the relief of pain from any of the following conditions:

1. Musculoskeletal trauma.

2. Burns.

3. Acute myocardial infarction.

4. Kidney stones.

5. Labor *prior* to crowning.

6. Other problems as defined by local EMS system.

It is not a supplement to other pain medications.

Contraindications

The following conditions or situations are contraindications to the use of nitrous oxide:

1. Shock.

2. Major facial injury.

3. Acute pulmonary edema, as 100% oxygen is needed.

4. Abdominal trauma or distension.

5. Known pneumothorax.

6. Chronic obstructive airway disease.

7. Any altered state of consciousness.

Precautions

The patient must not be assisted in holding the mask to his or her face, since inability to keep the mask on the face represents the point at which it should be stopped temporarily. By assisting the patient, the paramedic can increase the anesthesia effect beyond safe limits.

If the paramedic feels light-headed, the gas should be turned off, as judgment will be affected. Patient pain is preferable to paramedic ineffectiveness.

The nitrous oxide must be kept locked up since abuse by users has been a problem on occasion. Irreversible neurological damage from chronic abuse has been reported among licensed professionals. Some EMS systems limit nitrous oxide to age 10 or

above. This should be discussed with local EMS physicians.

Complications

Patient nausea and vomiting is one potential side effect which is individual and hard to predict. Patient drowsiness and light-headedness is common and a problem only if the patient becomes aggressive or combative.

EQUIPMENT

In the United States, nitrous oxide and oxygen are supplied as Nitronox. This consists of two cylinders—one containing oxygen, the other nitrous oxide—and a valve that provides a 50:50 mixture of the two gases (Figure 5.63). A mixture above 50% nitrous oxide is dangerous; 100% nitrous oxide deprives the patient of oxygen and is lethal.

The mixture of gases is piped to a demand valve to be held by the patient for self-administration to control pain. The tight face seal of the mask allows the patient to trigger the demand valve with inhalation. As the patient gets drowsy, the mask falls away from the patient's face but does not leak gases.

SKILL SEQUENCE

The skill sequence is divided into the four parts: confirming the order, preparing the medication, administering the medication, and confirming medication administration. The nickname "laughing gas" underestimates the potency of the medication; this formality is required for everyone's safety.

Confirm the Order

The paramedic needs to obtain an order for nitrous oxide after presenting a patient re-

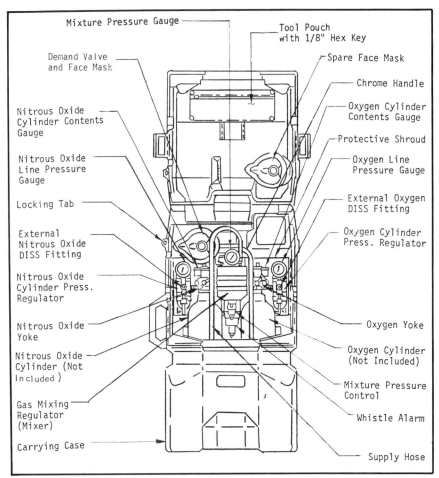

Figure 5-63 Schematic diagram of Nitronox system

port to base control personnel. The indications and contraindications are weighed at both ends of this communication.

Prepare the Medication

The nitrous oxide unit is best prepared before the shift in which it might be used. Both the oxygen and nitrous oxide tanks need to have adequate pressure. The valve needs to move to 50% but protect from higher concentrations of nitrous oxide. The demand valve and mask need to be clean to allow proper exhalation when applied to the face.

Administer the Medication

The patient is instructed on the purpose and method of administration and is told to expect to be drowsy and to use the mask only as needed to take the edge off the pain. As always, allergies should be rechecked.

Confirm Medication Administration

The paramedic should report the administration of the nitrous oxide and the patient response—both vital signs and level of consciousness.

SKILL PROFICIENCY TESTING

Skill Subcutaneous Injection (Figure 5.64)

Performance Demonstrate how to administer 0.2 cc of 1:1000 adrenalin (simulated) using an ampule and tuberculin syringe.

Conditions
1. Fellow student as simulated patient (an orange is acceptable but not preferred).

2. Ampule of water or saline labeled for the test as "Adrenalin—1 cc—1:1000" and other ampules.

3. 2 × 2 gauze in sterile wrapper.

4. Alcohol sponge.

5. Simulated radio or phone and drug box.

6. Evaluator explains that rescuer has just received an order to administer 0.3 or 0.2 cc (see above) subcutaneously to a teenager with asthma.

Standard
1. Rescuer follows the sequence in the Detailed Subcutaneous Medication Administration Guide, missing only 6 of the 29 steps. ☐

2. Time limit: 3 minutes. ☐

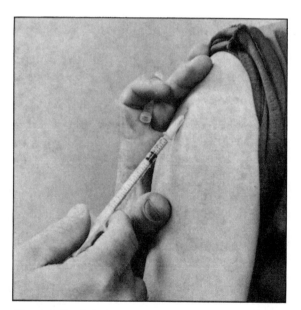

Figure 5–64

Student's Name _____ Date _____ Evaluator _____

Pass/Fail

SKILL PROFICIENCY TESTING

Skill   Intramuscular Injection (Figure 5.65)

Performance   Demonstrate how to inject 5 mg of morphine intramuscularly using a Tubex or similar preload.

Conditions

1. For testing purposes students may inject each other in the deltoid or use an injection manikin.

2. Tubex Tamp-R-Tel package with saline cartridge–needle units.

3. Tubex syringe.

4. Alcohol sponge.

5. Drug box.

6. Evaluator informs rescuer that he has just received an order to give 5 mg of morphine IM to a patient with a simulated tibia fracture.

Standard

1. Rescuer follows the sequence in the Detailed Intramuscular Medication Administration Guide, missing only 6 of the 30 steps.   ☐

2. Time limit: 3 minutes.   ☐

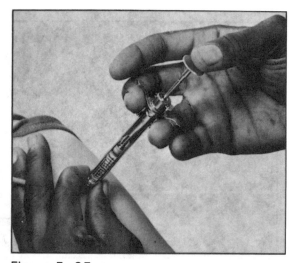

Figure 5-65

Student's Name _____ Date _____ Evaluator _____

Pass/Fail

SKILL PROFICIENCY TESTING

Skill Intravenous Preload Bolus Administration (Figure 5.66)

Performance Demonstrate how to administer 100 mg of lidocaine by IV bolus using a preloaded syringe.

Conditions

1. A manikin IV arm will be prepared in advance with a medical IV secured in place.

2. A preload syringe of lidocaine filled with water will be available to the student. Other syringes with water will also be available.

3. Alcohol sponge should be available.

4. The evaluator will explain that the rescuer has just received an order to give 100 mg of lidocaine by IV bolus for this simulated patient with a myocardial infarction (MI).

Standard

1. Rescuer follows the sequence in the Detailed Intravenous Bolus Medication Administration Guide, missing only 5 of the 26 steps. ☐

2. Time limit: 3 minutes. ☐

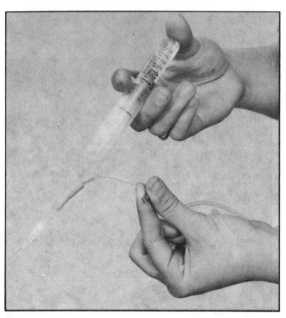

Figure 5–66

Student's Name _____ Date _____ Evaluator _____

Pass/Fail

SKILL PROFICIENCY TESTING

Skill   Intravenous Piggyback Drip (Figure 5.67)

Performance   Demonstrate how to administer a lidocaine IV piggyback drip.

Conditions   1. A manikin IV arm will be prepared in advance with a medical IV secured in place.

2. A simulated preload lidocaine syringe of 2 g of lidocaine will be available. The syringe will actually be filled with saline for safety.

3. The equipment for a second medical IV will be connected and aseptically capped.

4. A No. 22 needle will be available as well as an alcohol sponge, tape, and drug kit.

5. The evaluator will explain that the rescuer has just received an order to give 4 mg/min of lidocaine by IV piggyback drip.

Standard   1. Rescuer follows the sequence in the Detailed Intravenous Piggyback Medication Administration Guide, missing only 5 of the 24 steps.   ☐

2. Time limit: 3 minutes.   ☐

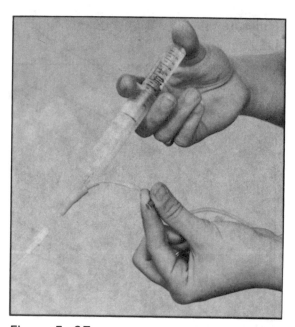

Figure 5-67

Student's Name _____ Date _____ Evaluator _____

Pass/Fail

SKILL PROFICIENCY TESTING

Skill   Inhalation Analgesia

Performance   Demonstrate how to administer a 50%/50% mixture of nitrous oxide and oxygen.

Conditions   1. Nitrous oxide equipment.

2. Attached demand valve.

3. Evaluate state of patient in severe pain from fractured tibia.

4. Blood pressure cuff and stethoscope.

Standard   1. Rescuer follows sequence in Detailed Inhalation Analgesia Guide, missing only 2 of 8 steps.   ☐

Student's Name _____ Date _____ Evaluator _____

Pass/Fail

6

Dysrhythmias

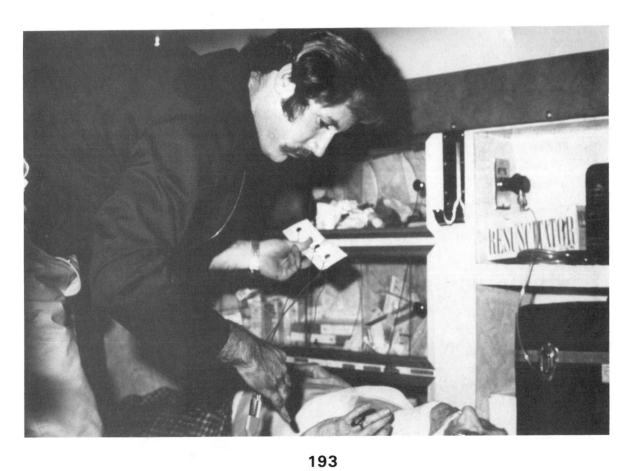

Skills Objectives

- **Monitoring**—Demonstrate how to apply monitor electrodes to a patient to obtain a lead II or MCL_1 oscilloscope reading and then a paper readout from a strip recorder.

- **Rhythm Recognition**—Demonstrate how to recognize dysrhythmias from a scope, paper, and slides.

- **Carotid Sinus Massage**—Demonstrate how to perform carotid massage on a patient with a symptomatic supraventricular tachycardia.

- **Two-Minute CPR**—Demonstrate how to perform 2 minutes of basic CPR using both single- and two-rescuer techniques on a Recording Anne.

- **Defibrillation**—Demonstrate how to check a defibrillator, evaluate a patient for ventricular fibrillation, and defibrillate correctly when indicated.

- **Automatic Defibrillation**—Demonstrate how to utilize an automatic defibrillator when monitoring is unavailable.

- **Non-Invasive External Pacing**—Demonstrate how to utilize an external pacemaker device for treating asystole.

Outline

Dysrhythmia Skills Description

Application of Monitor
  Electrodes
Paper Readout
Rhythm Interpretation
Carotid Sinus Massage
Two-Minute CPR
Defibrillation
Cardioversion
Pacemaker Magnet
Non-invasive External Pacing

Skill Proficiency Testing

Introduction
Special Considerations

Judgment
Equipment
Skill Sequence
Lab Practice

Dysrhythmia Skills Description

INTRODUCTION

Although dysrhythmias may occur secondarily to many types of stress on the heart, in the setting of a myocardial infarction (MI), if recognized early in the warning stage, many rhythms may be treated and lethal rhythms prevented. The paramedic must develop a logical approach to chest pain, beginning with a good advanced patient evaluation, and leading to a conclusion as to whether or not a patient might be having an

MI. Once this is suspected, analyzing the rhythm and watching for changes becomes an important task.

The skills then become the following:

1. Obtain a rhythm both on the oscilloscope and paper readout.

2. Interpret the rhythm correctly.

3. Select therapy (see therapy text).

4. Perform proper skills when indicated.

SPECIAL CONSIDERATIONS

Some principles to remember when treating dysrhythmias are the following:

1. Treat patients, not rhythms.

2. Pulse is a better guide to heart mechanical functions than is rhythm.

3. An alert patient with ventricular fibrillation on the monitor means artifact, or lead problems.

4. Advanced life-support skills are useless in cardiac arrest unless basic life support is started early and done well.

5. Cardiac arrest in trauma is hypovolemia until proven otherwise.

6. Exhaustion is a good reason to stop CPR (avoids increasing the number of patients).

7. Drugs given during cardiac arrest must be circulated by CPR to be effective.

Monitoring

The heart is a muscular pump controlled by recurring electrical impulses. Although the peripheral pulse is the best guide of the actual pumping effectiveness of the heart, monitoring a patient gives us insight into the electrical events triggering the pump. Heart

impulses may be monitored at the surface of the skin by monitor leads.

The full electrocardiogram employs five leads, one to each limb, as well as a moving chest lead. It therefore requires five leads to produce a full 12-lead electrocardiogram. The full electrocardiogram gives us information as to heart chamber size and the location of myocardial infarctions.

With the advent of coronary care units, the advantage of monitoring patients and treating warning arrhythmias before they turned into lethal arrhythmias (asystole and ventricular fibrillation) has become evident. Nurses are given special training in rhythm recognition and also given standing orders for rapid treatment. Often the abnormal rhythm is completely eliminated before the physician is notified.

The goal of putting monitor leads on a patient is to get a rhythm pattern to appear on an oscilloscope or on a paper strip. Rather than use the 12 leads of a full EKG (electrocardiogram—designed to check for heart attacks, chamber enlargement, etc.), the monitor uses three leads: positive, negative, and ground. A positive deflection or upward line is generated when the heart conduction goes toward the positive lead. The two most common locations for such leads are lead II and lead MCL$_1$ (Figures 6.1 and 6.2). Lead

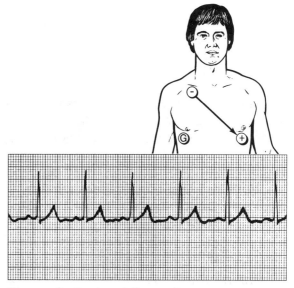

Figure 6-1 Lead II monitor.

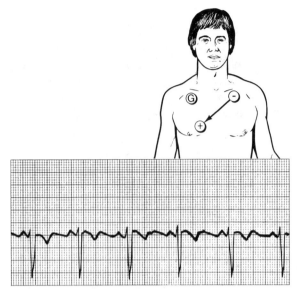

Figure 6–2   Lead MCL₁ monitor.

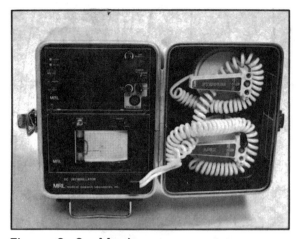

Figure 6–3   Monitor.

II is best for separating P waves from QRSs, and MCL₁ is best for checking ectopic beats.

A rhythm strip only needs to be 6 inches long to diagnose most rhythms. At normal paper speed, this takes 6 seconds. This should be the standard length of a rhythm strip when sent from the field to the base hospital unless a longer strip is requested. This avoids tying up the radio channel uselessly.

SKILL SEQUENCE

A certified paramedic can generally apply monitor electrodes within an EMS system without obtaining prior permission because it is not an invasive skill. (However, because these monitors generally also include defibrillators and therefore have some dangers, they should not be used by uncertified personnel.)

1. Rescuer reassures patient and then turns on the portable monitor to allow warm-

EQUIPMENT

A variety of portable monitors are available on the market. They are usually combined with the features of paddle readout, defibrillation, synchronized cardioversion, and paper strip recorder to be described later. Because the particular devices are capable of defibrillation, they are often simply referred to as defibrillators (Figure 6.3). Almost all of them have a place for a monitor cable to be plugged in. This in turn leads to the display of a rhythm on the oscilloscope screen.

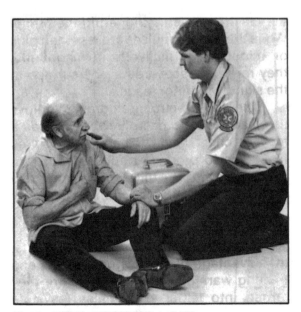

Figure 6–4   Reassure patient.

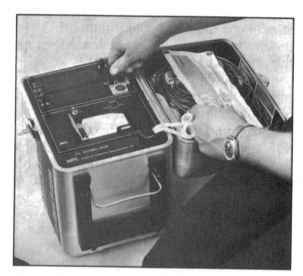

Figure 6-5   Turn on monitor.

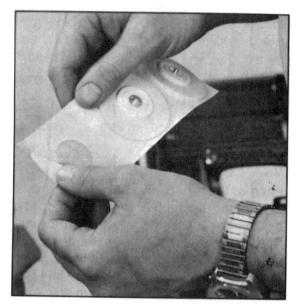

Figure 6-7   Prepare adhesive pad.

up time while leads are being applied to the chest (Figures 6.4 and 6.5).

2. Selects the lead used in the local EMS system: for example, lead II. Obtains patient cable (Figure 6.6).

3. Cleanses the skin. A number of monitor pads have their own small abrasive scrub brush and even soap for cleaning the skin. If these are present, they should be used appropriately (Figure 6.7).

4. Places the adhesive monitoring pads appropriately. For example, to create

a lead II, the paramedic should place the negative electrode just below or just above the right clavicle near the shoulder. The ground electrode is similarly placed near the left clavicle. The positive electrode is placed in the fifth intercostal space on the left anterior axillary line (Figure 6.8).

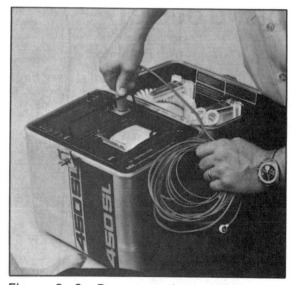

Figure 6-6   Prepare patient cable.

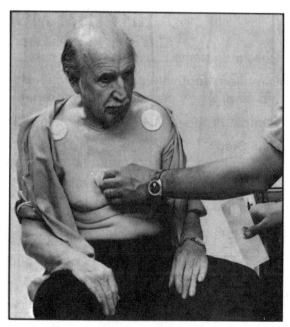

Figure 6-8   Apply monitor pad.

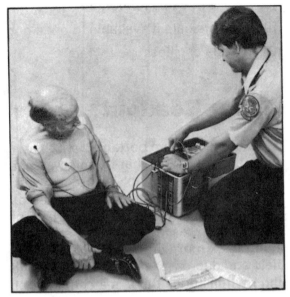

Figure 6–9   Observe monitor.

5. Snaps on the electrodes from a cable, correctly aligning positive, negative, and ground.

6. Plugs the cable into the monitor.

7. Adjusts the gain control so that a reasonably high complex is produced, further demonstrating P waves if present (Figure 6.9).

Reading the rhythm from the oscilloscope is discussed in a different section.

LAB PRACTICE

The following Rhythm Monitoring Guide has been prepared to aid in lab practice of this skill. Students can work in pairs. The evaluator will be the patient who is monitored.

RHYTHM MONITORING GUIDE

Rescuer's Name _____ Date _____ Evaluator _____

Directions for Evaluator: Place a check beside each item whenever an exam step is omitted, performed improperly, or presented improperly.

Sample Problem: A 45-year-old male with chest pain needs rhythm monitoring.

Step	Evaluation
1. Rescuer reassures patient as to the need for monitoring.	_____
2. Turns on monitor to allow warm-up time.	_____
3. Selects lead to be used when available on machine.	_____
4. Obtains patient cable.	_____
5. Opens monitor pads.	_____
6. Cleanses skin using abrasive brush if available.	_____
7. Applies adhesive monitoring pads appropriately.	_____
8. Snaps on electrodes from a patient cable, correctly aligning negative, positive, and ground positions.	_____
9. Plugs in cable to monitor.	_____
10. Adjusts gain if available to get a good-size display.	_____
11. Reads oscilloscope rhythm.	_____

Paper Readout

Most of the current portable defibrillators have the option of a paper readout from a strip recorder, which means that the rhythm can be written out on normal electrocardiograph paper. This option increases the paramedic's ability to bring back more of the material from the field and decreases the necessity of sending rhythms once there is a certain confidence between the paramedic and the base hospital.

EQUIPMENT

Each of the four or five brands of portable defibrillators, which have paper readout as an option place the electrocardiograph paper in a different location. Some of them allow the student to adjust the height or gain, while others have an automatic gain control which delivers a uniform display. In most cases once the gain has been set for the day, the operation of the paper readout simply involves pushing one button on and off.

SKILL SEQUENCE

The advanced rescuer must become very familiar with the equipment, and certainly it is important in this case to know how to change the electrocardiograph paper. It will therefore be part of this skill to put a paper roll into the paper readout section of the monitor defibrillator as well as to obtain a 6-second rhythm strip. The specific steps are as follows:

1. The student will be given a paper readout device which does not have paper in it. He or she will first have to open the paper readout mechanism.

2. Remove the paper from the nearby box and place it appropriately in the paper holder (Figure 6.10).

3. Then turn on the readout to make

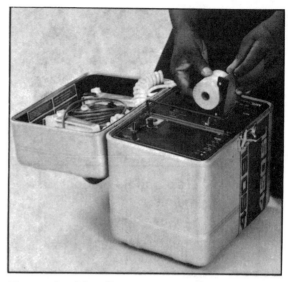

Figure 6–10   Put on new roll of paper.

sure the paper is running properly (Figures 6.11 to 6.13).

4. Turn it off again while the student makes sure there is an appropriate rhythm displayed on the oscilloscope screen.

5. Once rhythm appears to be appropriate the rescuer will then turn on the rhythm strip for 6 seconds, turn it off, and obtain the rhythm paper.

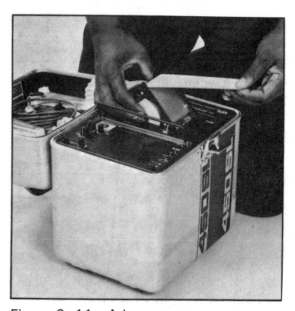

Figure 6–11   Advance paper.

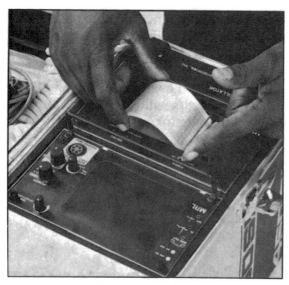

Figure 6-12   Close paper chamber.

LAB PRACTICE

The Paper Readout Procedure Guide is included as a student aid in the practice of this skill. The skill includes the addition of a new roll of rhythm strip paper to the monitor. The skill concludes with the production of a rhythm strip using paddles on the rescuer's own palms (Figure 6.14). Students work in pairs, with the second student being the evaluator.

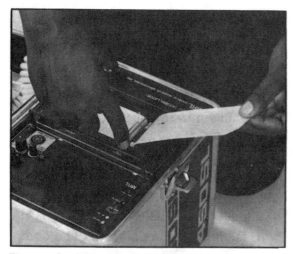

Figure 6-13   Push paper readout

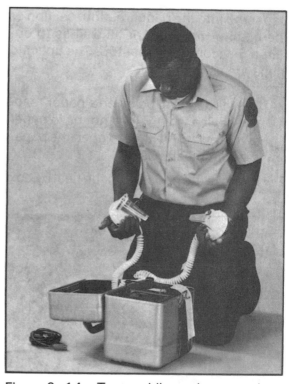

Figure 6-14   Test paddle readout on palms.

PAPER READOUT PROCEDURE GUIDE

Rescuer's Name _____ Date _____ Evaluator _____

Directions for Evaluator: Place a check beside each item whenever an exam step is omitted, performed improperly, or presented improperly.

	Step	**Evaluation**
1.	Rescuer opens paper roll compartment.	_____
2.	Obtains new roll of paper.	_____
3.	Sets roll into compartment.	_____
4.	Advances paper.	_____
5.	Closes paper compartment.	_____
6.	Pushes paper readout button.	_____
7.	Uses paddles on palms to get a complex.	_____
8.	Turns off paper readout button.	_____

Rhythm Recognition

This skill is taught in all standard theory texts. However, as a brief review the following comments are made. This section should be practiced *after* the rhythm course has been taught.

JUDGMENT

The skill is noninvasive and has no contraindications except where it delays care (e.g., in trauma it is seldom needed and may waste valuable time).

EQUIPMENT

For testing purposes rhythm can be presented in slides, paper strips, or on monitor screens. A number of simulators are on the market.

SKILL SEQUENCE

1. Always determine underlying rhythm first before looking at bizarre sections.

2. Determine atrial activity ("cherchez la P") and rate.

3. Determine QRS width, regularity, rate, and thus activity.

4. Determine relationship of P to QRS.

5. Give descriptive answer and conclusion.

LAB PRACTICE

The following rhythms are presented for practice. This skill is later tested using slides, rhythm strips on paper, and oscilloscope displays. Students may supply treatment choices if this has been presented in the parallel theory course.

Practice Rhythm Strips

NAME _____

DATE _____

Identify the following dysrhythmias and give initial treatment—including drug dosages and route of administration. All patients have possible MIs, and have O₂ and a medical IV (500 cc of D₅W) established.

1. A 46-year-old male with alcohol (ETOH) withdrawal; temperature 101 °F; blood pressure 130/90 (Figure 6.15)

    Diagnosis: _____

    Treatment: _____

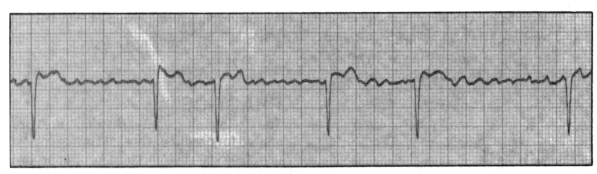

Figure 6–15

2. A 60-year-old female is dizzy and diaphoretic; blood pressure 90/60; palpable pulse (Figure 6.16)

    Diagnosis: _____

    Treatment: _____

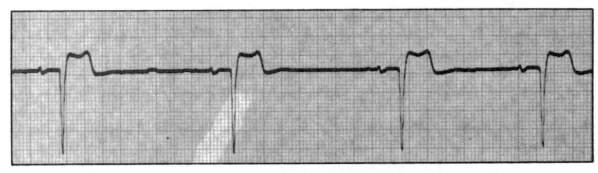

Figure 6–16

3. A 76-year-old male diabetic with cardiac history fell to the ground while working in the yard; responds to shaking; blood pressure 100/60 (Figure 6.17)

Diagnosis: _____

Treatment: _____

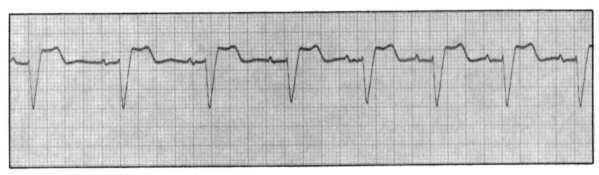

Figure 6-17

4. An 80-year-old female; asymptomatic; blood pressure 110/80 (Figure 6.18)

Diagnosis: _____

Treatment: _____

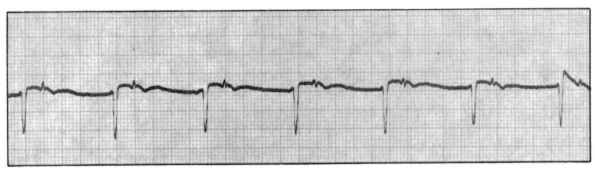

Figure 6-18

5. A 58-year-old male fainted; blood pressure 40/0 (Figure 6.19)

Diagnosis: _____

Treatment: _____

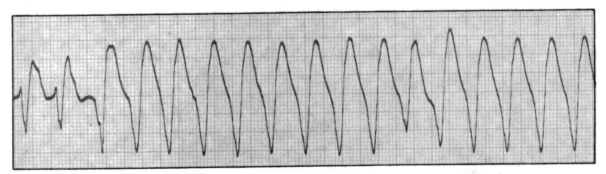

Figure 6-19

6. Patient is asymptomatic (Figure 6.20)

Diagnosis: _____

Treatment: _____

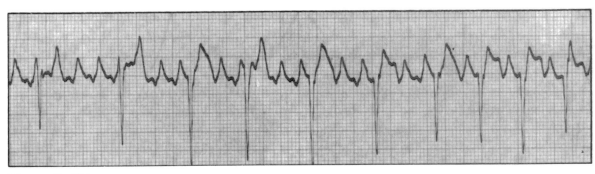

Figure 6-20

7. Patient having acute MI (Figure 6.21)

Diagnosis: _____

Treatment: _____

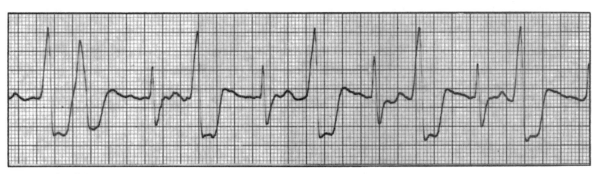

Figure 6-21

8. Patient is symptomatic; has a feeling of pounding in his chest (Figure 6.22)

Diagnosis: _____

Treatment: _____

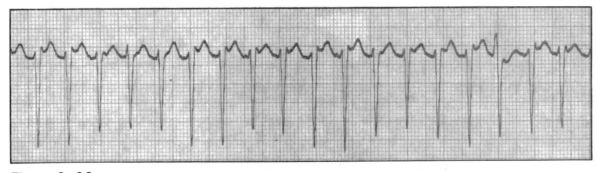

Figure 6-22

9. A 60-year-old male; unresponsive; absence of pulse and respirations (Figure 6.23)

Diagnosis: _____

Treatment: _____

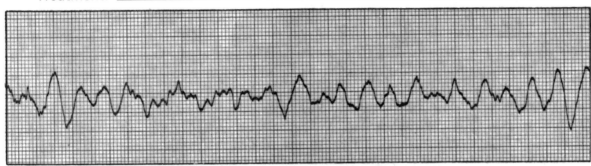

Figure 6–23

10. A 50-year-old male; awake, alert, and oriented; no complaints of chest pain; blood pressure 100/60 (Figure 6.24)

Diagnosis: _____

Treatment: _____

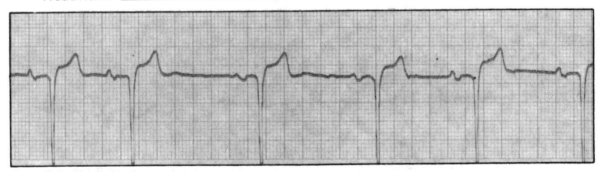

Figure 6–24

11. A 70-year-old male; diaphoretic with decreasing level of consciousness; blood pressure 90/50 (Figure 6.25)

Diagnosis: _____

Treatment: _____

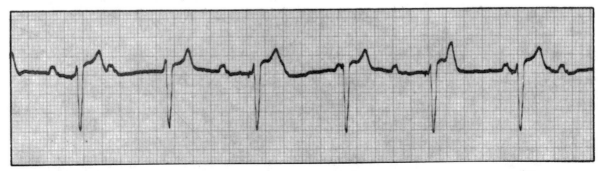

Figure 6–25

12. A 50-year-old male; blood pressure 120/70, respiration 24 (Figure 6.26)

Diagnosis: _____

Treatment: _____

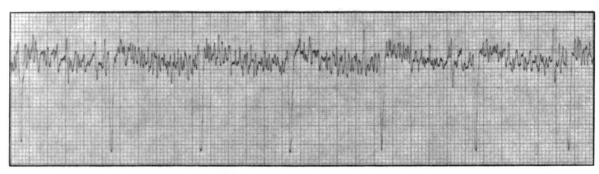

Figure 6-26

13. A 60-year-old male; patient is unresponsive and diaphoretic; unable to obtain blood pressure, no palpable pulse (Figure 6.27)

Diagnosis: _____

Treatment: _____

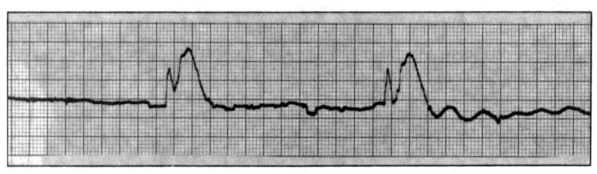

Figure 6-27

14. A 65-year-old male; blood pressure 130/70, pulse 60, respiration 20; patient is awake and alert; no chest pain (Figure 6.28)

Diagnosis: _____

Treatment: _____

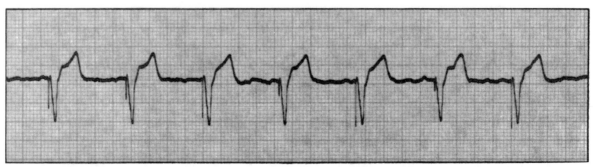

Figure 6-28

15. A 40-year-old male; blood pressure 120/70, respiration 20 (heart rate normally 50–60);
complaints of substernal chest pain (Figure 6.29)

Diagnosis: _____

Treatment: _____

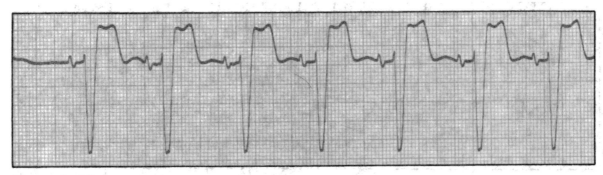

Figure 6–29

16. A 60-year-old male; blood pressure 170/90, pulse 60, respiration 32 (Figure 6.30)

Diagnosis: _____

Treatment: _____

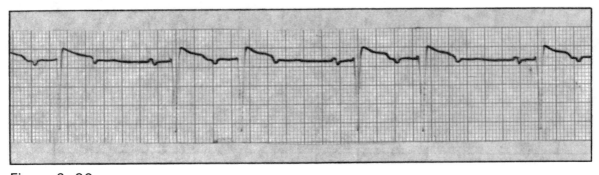

Figure 6–30

17. A 65-year-old male; cyanotic; no pulse (Figure 6.31)

Diagnosis: _____

Treatment: _____

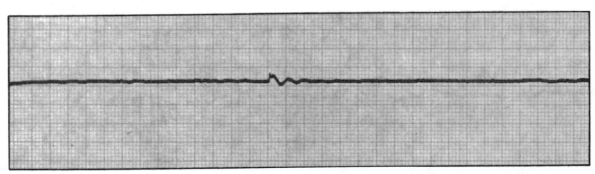

Figure 6–31

18. A 70-year-old male; dizzy; blood pressure 90/70 (Figure 6.32)

Diagnosis: _____

Treatment: _____

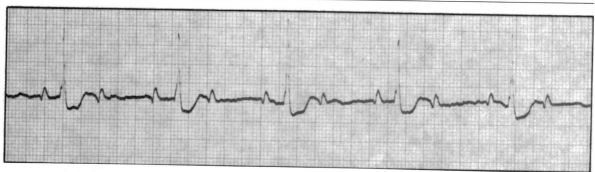

Figure 6-32

19. A 70-year-old male with chest pain; blood pressure 90/60, respiration 24; patient alert (Figure 6.33)

Diagnosis: _____

Treatment: _____

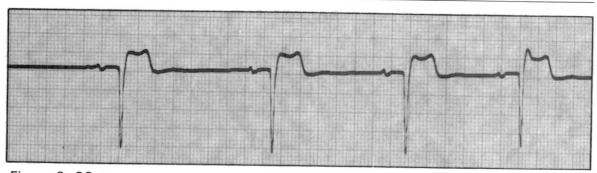

Figure 6-33

20. An 80-year-old male; blood pressure 90/60; patient confused and diaphoretic (Figure 6.34)

Diagnosis: _____

Treatment: _____

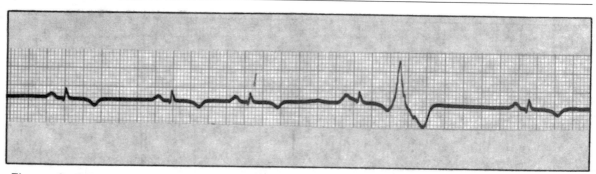

Figure 6-34

Rhythm Answers

Note: For treatment, check with instructor.

1. Atrial fibrillation (with good ventricular response)

2. Sinus bradycardia, symptomatic

3. Normal sinus rhythm

4. Normal or junctional rhythm

5. Ventricular tachycardia

6. Atrial tachycardia (with variable conduction)

7. Ventricular bigeminy

8. Supraventricular tachycardia

9. Ventricular fibrillation

10. First-degree heart block/sinus arrhythmia

11. Third-degree heart block

12. 60-Cycle artifact

13. Agonal or ideoventricular rhythm

14. Pacemaker rhythm, capturing

15. Normal sinus rhythm

16. Second-degree AV block—Mobitz I (Wenkebach)

17. Asystole

18. Second-degree AV block—Mobitz II

19. Sinus bradycardia with first-degree AV block

20. Sinus bradycardia with a premature ventricular contraction

Treatments still vary and should be defined by instructors. Thus treatment options are not given in this book.

Carotid Sinus Massage

The supraventricular tachcardia dysrhythmia can often be stopped if the vagus nerve is stimulated. Many techniques are used to stimulate the vagus nerve. The first usually tried is breath holding plus bearing down, called the Valsalva maneuver. A second, recently discovered technique involves placing a patient's face in ice water for 15 seconds, or alternative a cold wet cloth. This stimulates the diving reflex, which slows the pulse. A third maneuver is carotid sinus massage. When these maneuvers are unsuccessful, a variety of drugs may be used. Carotid sinus massage (CSM) is usually the limit to which vagal stimulation is undertaken by paramedics in the prehospital setting. Some experts call the skill carotid sinus pressure (CSP) emphasizing pressure over massage.

JUDGMENT

Indications

Carotid sinus massage is indicated in the patient with paroxysmal supraventricular tachycardia which is symptomatic (producing dyspnea or dizziness)

Contraindications

Carotid sinus massage is contraindicated in the patient with known carotid artery disease or known stroke history or the absence of carotid pulse on one side or bruiets (turbulance) heard with stethoscope when ausculated over artery.

Precautions

The rescuer should take the precaution of performing carotid sinus massage while the patient is monitored so that the possibility of asystole is carefully evaluated. An IV line should be in place and O₂ flowing.

Complications

The following complications can occur:

1. Temporary or prolonged asystole as well as other dysrhythmias may occur.

2. Theoretically, a stroke could occur with carotid artery pressure—consider performing on patient's dominent side so that if stroke occurs, patient has use of dominant hand.

EQUIPMENT

Carotid sinus massage requires no equipment other than having the patient monitored during the procedure with an IV of D₅W O₂ running.

SKILL SEQUENCE

The rescuer begins by confirming that the patient has a symptomatic supraventricular tachycardia unresponsive to the Valsalva maneuver. He or she continues to monitor patient throughout procedure and has administered O₂ and medical IVs in place.

The base hospital orders carotid sinus massage. The rescuer explains to the patient that he or she will be rubbing the patient's neck in order to slow down the patient's pulse. The rescuer first checks each carotid pulse and checks for carotid bruiets. He feels the carotid pulse near the angle of the jaw on one side with head turned to the other (Figure 6.35). The rescuer rubs the carotid artery with two fingers vertically back and forth while watching the oscilloscope monitor for 10 to 15 seconds (Figure 6.36). (Alternatively, rapid, firm, direct pressure on the sinus is recommended by many.) Stop after 10 to 15 seconds, or at the first sign of a decreased heart rate!

The rescuer obtains a rhythm strip before, during, and after the procedure in order to inform the base hospital what has

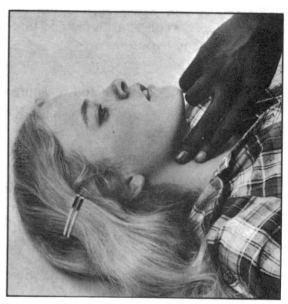

Figure 6–35   Find carotid sinus area.

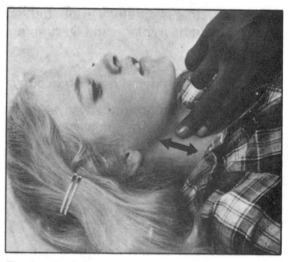

Figure 6–36   Massage carotid sinus.

occurred. The rescuer may repeat after 2 to 3 minutes on the same or opposite side. He or she does not massage both carotid arteries at the same time.

LAB PRACTICE

The following Carotid Sinus Massage Procedure Guide is provided to aid in lab practice of this skill. The skill should be tried on a manikin, as many people are very sensitive to massage and can become asystolic. Students work in pairs, with one student as rescuer and the other as evaluator.

CAROTID SINUS MASSAGE PROCEDURE GUIDE

Rescuer's Name _____ Date _____ Evaluator _____

Directions for Evaluator: Place a check beside each item whenever an exam step is omitted, performed improperly, or presented improperly.

Sample Patient Problem: A 24-year-old female with recurrent episodes of supraventricular tachycardia. This episode has lasted 2 hours, does not respond to Valsalva maneuvers, and is very dizzy and hypotensive.

Step	Evaluation
1. Rescuer introduces self and reassures.	_____
2. Makes sure that patient is monitored, has oxygen going, and has a D_5W IV in place.	_____
3. Explains procedure.	_____
4. Checks each carotid artery for pulse and bruiets.	_____
5. Feels carotid sinus on right with head turned to left.	_____
6. Massages carotid sinus for 10 to 15 seconds while watching monitor.	_____
7. Obtains a rhythm strip before, during, and after.	_____
8. Repeats procedure on other side if told that the dysrhythmia persists.	_____
9. Does not massage both sides at once.	_____
10. Informs base hospital of results.	_____

Two-Minute CPR

The following cardiopulmonary resuscitation steps are taught at the basic life-support level:

1. Infant CPR

2. Single-rescuer CPR

3. Two-rescuer CPR

4. Moving CPR

It is expected at the basic level that a rescuer can also use an adjunct such as a demand valve and maintain good CPR.

The advanced rescuer must be expert at these basic skills. To demonstrate such expertise he is expected to perform single-rescuer CPR, move into two-rescuer CPR, and switch places with the other rescuer in a continuous 2-minute sequence. The sequence is recorded on a recording tape.

JUDGMENT

Indications

As with all CPR, the indication is an unresponsive, apneic, pulseless patient. It is reasonable to start CPR when the pulse is so slow as to be nonperfusing. This occurs in the newborn below a rate of 60.

Contraindications

The absolute contraindications include rigor mortis, decapitation, and postmortem lividity. The more debated contraindications include an adult who is pulseless and apneic more than 10 minutes and a patient about to die of cancer.

Precautions

Rescuers should be sure to watch for the chest to rise during ventilation to avoid missing an airway obstruction. Proper hand posi-

tion avoids unnecessary chest trauma. The possibility of a spine injury trauma makes the jaw lift a preferred technique, but if a good airway is not obtained, other maneuvers are warranted.

Complications

The following complications can occur with CPR:

1. Gastric distension with vomiting and aspiration

2. Pneumothorax

3. Rib fracture or flail chest

4. Spleen or liver laceration

5. Cardiac muscle damage

6. Increasing internal bleeding

All of these are significant but should not deter the rescuer from doing CPR when indicated.

EQUIPMENT

The Laerdale Recording Anne remains the primary standard in the United States at this time. It must be operational, clean, and properly filled with recording paper to allow a continuous 2-minute strip. Some instructors have found it necessary to remove the arms of the manikin and lift the coat up to allow free running of the 2-minute tape without having the tape get caught in clothing.

SKILL SEQUENCE

The rescuer is given the problem that he or she is the first person on the scene where a patient has suddenly collapsed. The first rescuer arrives alone and performs 1-minute, single-rescuer CPR on a Recording Anne, matching all the criteria under single-rescuer CPR standards (Figures 6.37 and 6.38).

CARDIOPULMONARY RESUSCITATION

SINGLE RESCUER

15 COMPRESSIONS — 2 VENTILATIONS

Maintain a straight compression/relaxation line.

Do not allow lungs to deflate between ventilation.

Compressions 50% relaxation 50%.

Ventilation volume of at least .8 liters.

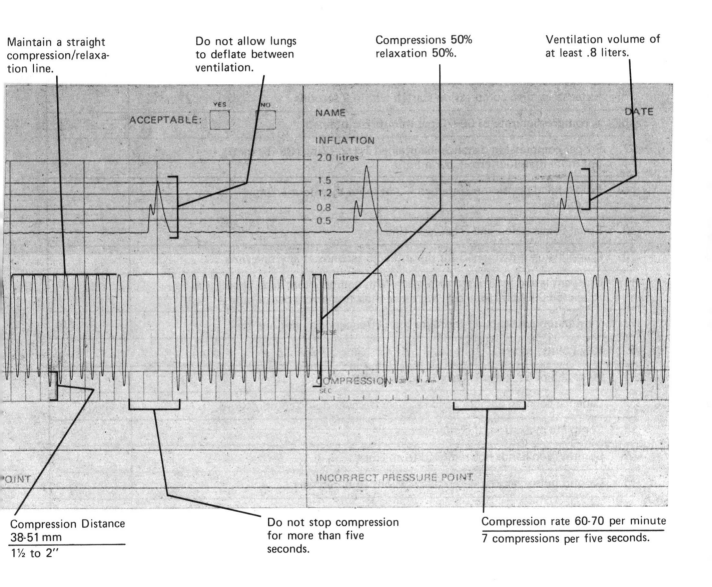

Compression Distance 38-51 mm
_____
1½ to 2″

Do not stop compression for more than five seconds.

Compression rate 60-70 per minute
_____
7 compressions per five seconds.

Figure 6–37   Single-rescuer CPR standards.

CARDIOPULMONARY RESUSCITATION

TWO RESCUERS

5 COMPRESSIONS — 1 VENTILATION

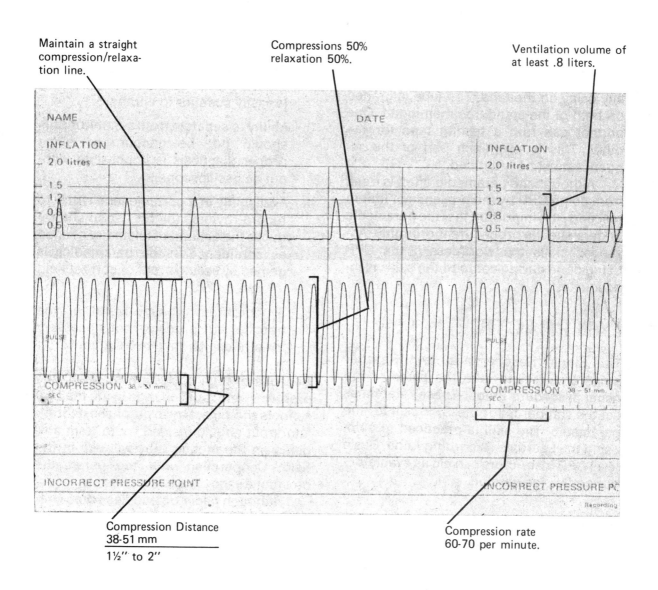

Maintain a straight compression/relaxation line.

Compressions 50% relaxation 50%.

Ventilation volume of at least .8 liters.

Compression Distance
38-51 mm
1½" to 2"

Compression rate 60-70 per minute.

Figure 6-38   Two-rescuer CPR standards.

SINGLE-RESCUER—ADULT

Name _____ Date _____

A. Performance Sequence	Maximum Elapsed Time (sec)	Single Rescuer: Adult
1. Unresponsiveness established within 10 seconds "Are you okay?" × 3	10	
2. Airway opened and breathing assessed within 5 seconds	15	
3. Initial two ventilations (1 to 1½ seconds per breath) allowing for exhalation between breaths	18	
4. Cardiac function assessed within 10 seconds— palpation of the carotid pulse for at least 5 seconds	28	
5. External cardiac compression started within 2 seconds	30	
6. A compression rate of 80 to 100 maintained (achieving 54 to 66 per minute)		
7. Proper compression distance maintained (1½ to 2 in., 39 to 51 mm), with no more than four errors per minute		
8. Proper hand position maintained, with no more than four errors per minute		
9. Equal compression and relaxation time		
10. Compression not stopped for more than 7 seconds at any one time		
11. Two ventilations interposed between each 15 compressions: a. each ventilation to exceed 0.8 liter b. allowing lungs to deflate between ventilations c. no ventilation to exceed 2 liters d. not allowing two errors per minute		

B. Key Points

1. Pulse status checked after 1 minute	
2. Complete relaxation of compressions	
3. Compression hand not removed from chest during relaxation	
4. Compression pressure applied straight downward	

Evaluator _____

Comments: _____

_____

_____

TWO-RESCUER — ADULT

Name _____ Date _____

A. Performance Sequence	Maximum Elapsed Time (sec)	Two Rescuer: Adult
1. Unresponsiveness established within 10 seconds "Are you okay?" × 3	10	
2. Airway opened and breathing assessed within 5 seconds	15	
3. Initial two ventilations (1 to 1½ seconds per breath) allowing for exhalation between breaths	18	
4. Cardiac function assessed within 10 seconds	28	
5. External cardiac compression started within 2 seconds	30	
6. A compression rate of 80 to 100 per minute maintained		
7. Proper compression distance maintained 1½ to 2 in. (39 to 51 mm); no more than four errors per minute		
8. Proper hand position maintained; no more than four errors per minute		
9. Equal compression and relaxation time		
10. Compression not stopped for more than 7 seconds at any one time		
11. One ventilation after each fifth compression; each ventilation to exceed 0.8 liter (800 cc); a pause is allowed between compression 5 and 1 so that there is complete lung inflation; no more than two errors per minute; no ventilation to exceed 2 liters		

B. Key Points		
1. Pulse and pulse status checked and rechecked		
2. Cadence counted audibly by rescuer doing compression (one and two and . . .)		
3. Complete relaxation of compressions		
4. Compression hands not removed from chest		
5. Carotid pulse checked with compressions		
6. Compression pressure applied straight down		
7. Carotid pulse checked without compression after 2 minutes		

Evaluator _____

Comments: _____

_____

_____

Defibrillation

As almost all of the survivors of cardiac arrest treated by paramedics turn out in retrospect to have had ventricular fibrillation, defibrillation is one of the most critical skills of the paramedic. Because improper use of the equipment can endanger the patient, the rescuer, and other rescuers, many precautions are taken to make sure that the skill is handled safely.

EQUIPMENT

All new defibrillators are of the direct current type since they are lighter, more portable, and more effective than the older alternating current type. They differ in some of the following features:

1. Maximum delivered watt/seconds of power to a 50 ohm resistance testor—all should be above 325 watt/seconds when fully charged.

2. The wave form of the discharge; but there is little proof that one wave form is vastly superior to another.

3. Ability to separate from a monitor (this should not be encouraged since proper diagnosis is impossible without an oscilloscope.)

4. Availability of a portable tape writer to record rhythms (highly useful and reduces the amount of telemetry needed as confidence in the paramedics is gained by seeing proof of correct field interpretation.)

5. Synchronizer option—more useful in the hospital but rarely necessary for prehospital rhythm treatment.

Because of high cost, high maintenance problems, and rapid change in the market, schools should not try to purchase defibrillators but should instead try to train students on the models they will use in the field. Cooperation with the paramedic provider agency is usually possible.

Although pediatric paddles come with some models, the adult paddles used anteroposteriorly (AP) work fine. Of course the energy setting would be much lower.

JUDGMENT

Indications

Defibrillation is indicated for ventricular fibrillation. Cardioversion, a more general term for changing the heart rhythm electrically, is indicated for any tachyarrhythmia causing severe shock. Intravenous medication is not indicated in the latter situation because severe shock impedes circulation of the medication.

Contraindications

The only contraindication for defibrillating ventricular fibrillation would be the presence of a factor that would cause injury to a paramedic or another patient; for example, if two patients were touching and could not be separated prior to defibrillation. Another example of potential injury might be the presence of a flammable gas such as gasoline vapor or ether vapor. Defibrillating in the rain may increase the chance of arcing to a paramedic. Oxygen supports combustion and should be pulled back during defibrillation.

Precautions

The following precautions must be taken during defibrillation:

1. Look to see that everyone hears the order, "CLEAR."

2. Disconnect the bag-valve resuscitator from the ET tube or EOA mask if they are in place.

3. No conductor can be touching anything that would lead to another person.

4. Make sure that there are no flammable gases in the area.

5. Make sure that there is no bridge of conduction gel between paddles to produce a skin bridge.

6. Make sure that the paddles are fully charged and well covered with conductive material.

7. Do not discharge paddles against each other in practice unless allowed by the manufacturer.

8. Make sure that the patient being defibrillated is pulseless and not just registering an artifact rhythm.

9. Make sure that the patient does not carry a loaded gun.

Complications

The following complications may occur:

1. Spark jumping to another rescuer, potentially causing a minor burn or even ventricular fibrillation

2. Some damage to the myocardial muscle mass

3. Skin bridging, causing chest wall arc

4. Poor skin contact, causing a burn

5. Tetanic contraction, causing loss of IV or other poorly attached equipment

6. Explosion if a flammable gas is present

SKILL SEQUENCE

Check the Equipment

The paramedic must take a number of steps to check the equipment. He or she must turn the defibrillator on and check for a low battery. Next he or she fully charges paddles and reads watt/seconds delivered when discharged through a testing unit.

The paramedic must check paddles for surface pitting or dry gel causing an uneven surface. He or she also makes sure that paddles do not discharge on a two-button system unless both buttons are pushed.

Obtain a Paddle Readout Rhythm

To obtain a paddle readout rhythm, the paramedic must make sure there is no charge on the paddles. He or she then uses a pair of gel pads on the chest of a manikin, placing one just below the right clavicle and the other at the apex of the heart.

Next the paramedic makes sure that the monitor cable is unplugged or the paddle switch is on so that the rhythm produced will be from the paddles. Then the paramedic checks the rhythm by applying the paddles. During the morning check of the rig, the paramedic can check the paddle readout by placing the switch to paddle and putting the paddles on the palms of the hand.

Defibrillate the Patient

The steps that must be followed to defibrillate the patient are important. The paramedic makes sure that the simulated patient is an unresponsive, apneic, pulseless patient (Figures 6.39 and 6.40). Next he or she makes sure that basic CPR is being done adequately. Then the paramedic makes sure that the gel pads are properly set on the chest (or lubricates the paddles; Figures

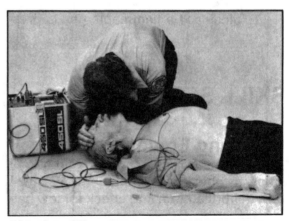

Figure 6–39   Confirm patient is apneic.

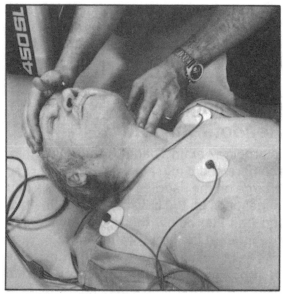

Figure 6–40   Confirm patient is pulseless. (Lead II)

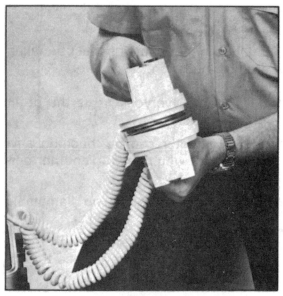

Figure 6–42   Rub paddles together.

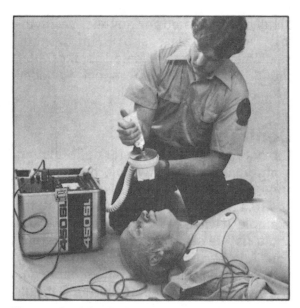

Figure 6–41   Lubricate defibrillation paddles.

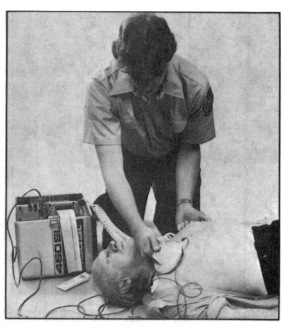

Figure 6–43   Apply paddles to check monitor.

6.41 and 6.42) and that the synchronizer button, if preset, is off.

Next the paramedic rechecks the paddle readout (Figures 6.43 and 6.44) and if ventricular fibrillation charges paddles to 200 joules initially, 200 to 300 for the second defibrillation, and full power for the third and subsequent defibrillations (Figure 6.45). Then after final ventilation the paramedic says, ''Stop CPR and clear.'' (Figure 6.46). He or she looks and checks that all rescuers are clear and then applies paddles

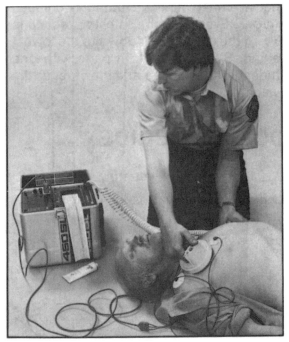

Figure 6-44   Obtain rhythm strip readout.

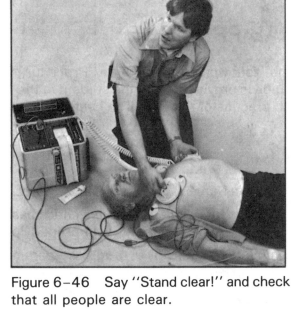

Figure 6-46   Say "Stand clear!" and check that all people are clear.

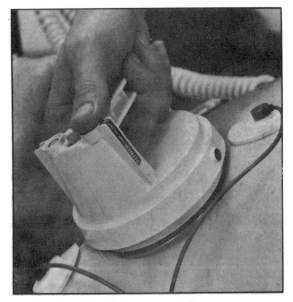

Figure 6-45   Charge paddles.

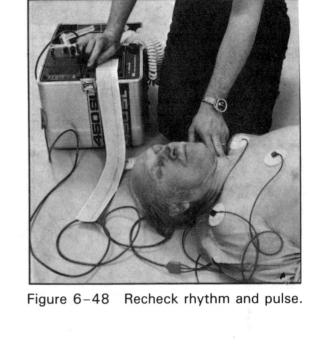

Figure 6-48   Recheck rhythm and pulse.

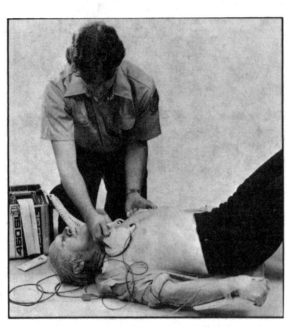

Figure 6-47   Discharge paddles.

with 20 to 25 pounds of force and defibrillates (Figure 6.47). It is good to run a paper readout just before, during, and after defibrillation to monitor the rhythm during this procedure.

The paramedic then leaves paddles on chest another 10 seconds to get a new rhythm reading (Figure 6.48). Next he or she removes paddles and resumes CPR, if no rhythm appears. If a rhythm appears, the paramedic immediately sees if it is producing a pulse. If a good pulse is present, he or she checks a blood pressure.

Successful defibrillation is usually preceded by oxygenation, epinephrine, and good CPR, and is followed by a bolus and then a drip of lidocaine. These steps are used in a full resuscitation.

LAB PRACTICE

The following Defibrillation Procedure Guide is provided to aid the student in lab practice of this skill. The best manikin for practice is the Recording Anne with the special chest plate including two metal buttons. Even then the safest approach is to turn the defibrillator down to the lowest setting. Students work in pairs, with one student as the rescuer and the other as the evaluator.

DEFIBRILLATION PROCEDURE GUIDE

Rescuer's Name _____ Date _____ Evaluator _____

Directions for Evaluator: Place a check beside each item whenever an exam step is omitted, performed improperly, or presented improperly.

Sample Patient Problem: CPR in progress—paramedic arrives with defibrillator.

Step	Method	Evaluation
1. Check the equipment (done during morning checkout)	a. The paramedic first turns on the defibrillator.	_____
	b. Looks for low battery.	_____
	c. Fully charges paddles.	_____
	d. Tests delivered energy on a 50-ohm resistance testor.	_____
	e. Checks paddle surfaces for pitting.	_____
2. Obtain the paddle readout	a. Checks to see that there is no charge on paddles.	_____
	b. Makes sure that the cable is not the input to the monitor.	_____
	c. Checks the rhythm by applying the paddles.	_____
	d. Interprets if ventricular fibrillation is present.	_____
3. Defibrillate the patient	a. Confirms that patient is unresponsive.	_____
	b. Confirms that patient is apneic and pulseless.	_____
	c. Makes sure that basic CPR is being done well with chest rising and pulse produced with compression.	_____
	d. Makes sure that synchronizer button is off.	_____
	e. Uses gel pads or gel paste for conduction.	_____
	f. Checks paddle conduction and position.	_____
	g. Charges paddles.*	_____
	h. Stops CPR, says "Stand clear," *and looks to see that all are clear.*	_____
	i. Applies paddles with 20 to 25 pounds of pressure.	_____
	j. Discharges paddles.	_____
	k. Obtains new paddle readout.	_____
	l. Removes paddles; if rhythm present, checks pulse.	_____

*For classroom safety the lowest power should be used.

Cardioversion

Cardioversion differs from defibrillation in that the defibrillator is set to recognize an R wave and thus avoids shocking a patient on the vulnerable part of the T wave.

Rhythm

The rhythms used for such conversion in the field are *highly* symptomatic (coma, unconsciousness, shock, or cyanosis) tachycardias: (1) ventricular tachycardia with a steady baseline; (2) supraventricular tachycardia with a very fast ventricular response.

Skill

The skill is not separately defined as if differs from defibrillation primarily in its indications and in pressing the synchronizer button. Note that a large Q or S wave can be made upright by reversing the + and − leads. A much lower watt/seconds of energy will be used starting at 50 joules.

Precautions

The synchronizer button must never be on when defibrillating ventricular fibrillation. Make sure that the machine does not sense a tall T wave and mistake it for an R wave.

LAB PRACTICE

There is no separate lab practice, guide, or skill test for this skill.

Pacemaker Magnet

With increasing numbers of patients having permanent pacemakers, dealing with pacemaker failure is becoming a frequent prehospital skill. Some of these patients can simply be transported to the hospital, others can be treated with drugs, and still others can be helped with the use of a special horseshoe magnet.

Although there are many types of pacemakers, for the purposes of this discussion the paramedic need only know about the most common pacemaker—the demand pacemaker. The pacemaker electrode is inserted either on the surface of the heart (epicardial—Figure 6.49) or in the right ventricle passed through a vein (endocardial—Figure 6.50). The pacemaker itself is placed beneath the skin of the chest wall.

The demand pacemaker is set to fire when the patient's own R wave is absent or delayed. It is on standby when the patient has a normal rhythm. This is why it is also called R-wave inhibited. An example of the demand pacemaker rhythm is displayed in Figure 6.51. The demand pacemaker can be changed with a magnet to a fixed mode in which the pacemaker fires regardless of the patient's rhythm.

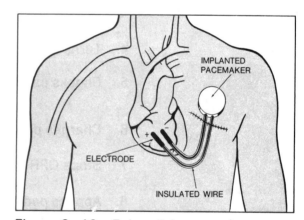

Figure 6–49   Epicardial pacemaker.

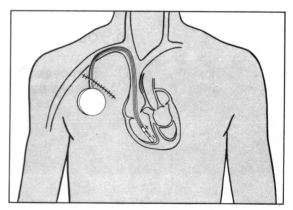

Figure 6–50   Endocardial pacemaker.

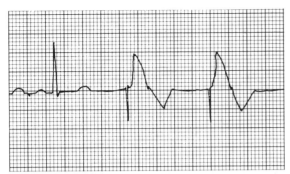

Figure 6–51   Demand pacemaker rhythm.

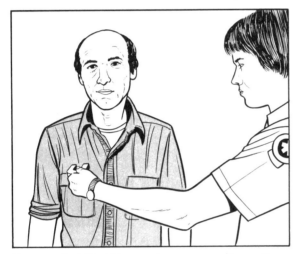

Figure 6–52   Horseshoe magnet application.

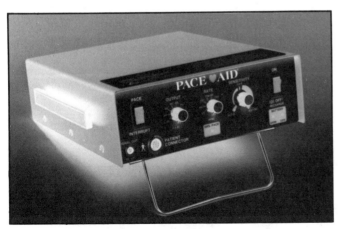

Figure 6–53   The Pace-Aid® 53.

The pacemaker may fail in several ways: (1) stop sensing the R wave; (2) stop capturing the ventricle; (3) speed up to become a runaway pacemaker. If the affected patient is very symptomatic due to a secondary sudden change in cardiac output, one treatment is to use a horseshoe magnet to change the demand mode to a fixed-mode operation.

The technique for using such a magnet would be: (1) remove bar from magnet staying at least 2 feet away from patient; (2) approach the pacemaker in the chest wall with the horseshoe magnet horizontal (Figure 6.52); (3) if the patient's rhythm turns to a fixed pacemaker rate and the patient improves, hold the magnet in place during transport; (4) if the patient's rhythm turns to a fixed pacemaker rate and the patient gets worse, remove the magnet; (5) if there is no change, remove the magnet 2 feet away, apply the bar, turn it over 180 degrees, remove the bar, and reapply to pacemaker. One special precaution is not to rotate the magnet near the patient.

This skill is unusual and dependent on the approval of the cardiologists in the EMS area being served. It is not included in the lab sessions or in the testing sessions. In the future it may become a routine paramedic skill, especially in areas serving retirement communities. The skill is not defined with a specific performance or test.

Noninvasive External Pacing

The ideal treatment of a severe bradycardia or asystole is the substitution of an electronic pacemaker to take over the function of the damaged conduction system of the heart (Figure 6.53). Until recently, this skill was largely confined to intravenously introduced internal pacemakers used in the intensive care units.

External pacing was done with limited success using needles—one placed through

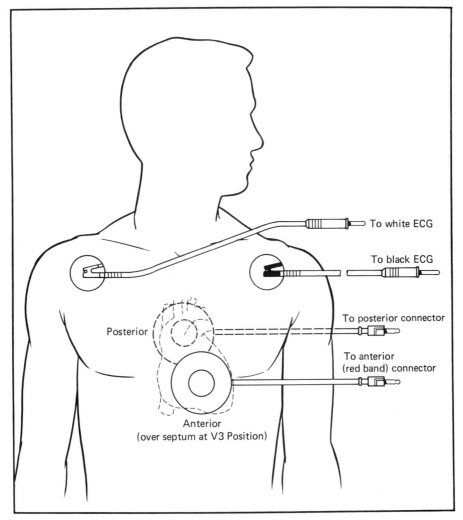

Figure 6–54   Applying external electrodes.

the heart muscle and hooked to hold on the endocardial surface and the other placed in the skin. The time of training when contrasted to the results has not been encouraging. Recently, the Federal Drug Administration has approved the use of external pacing from external anterior/posterior electrodes (Figure 6.54). The skill in this section is defined for one brand available called Pace-Aid.

The goal of a pacemaker is to send a large enough electrical signal to capture the heart and produce a coordinated contraction. When the heart regains its own rhythm in the demand mode, the pacemaker should sense this and shut off, being available only on demand. Thus a pacemaker has features such as capture, sensing, and demand features. An example of capture is shown in Figure 6.55.

JUDGMENT

Indications

External pacing is indicated for any patient who is unconscious and in severe shock or pulseless due to severe bradycardia or asystole, and unresponsive to the usual ACLS medications.

The two tracings shown below are from a patient successfully resuscitated by ambulance personnel in Brighton, England:

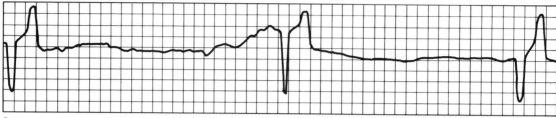

Spontaneous rhythm

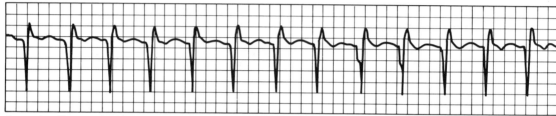

Pacemaker (front to back)

Figure 6-55

Contraindications

External pacing should not be used in the absence of training and certification by the local EMS authority operating under medical control.

Precautions

1. Only certified personnel may use external pacing.

2. Never use on a child less than 12 years of age since research in children has not been completed.

3. Check battery weekly and after each usage.

SKILL SEQUENCE

1. Begin CPR as normally indicated; then check cardiac rhythm.

2. Stop CPR and quickly attach anterior and posterior electrodes if rhythm is asystole.

3. Resume CPR for three cycles, then stop again.

4. Turn on external pacemaker.

5. If pacing light flashes, check carotid pulse.

6. If pulse, check blood pressure.

7. If apneic, give two ventilations for each 15 pacing cycles.

8. If no pulse, resume CPR and use ACLS meds as indicated, compressing patient at same time as pulsing jerk.

CONCLUSION

At least one-fourth of most paramedic classroom time during initial training is usually spent learning how to obtain, differentiate, and treat dysrhythmias. The skills involved are among the most important of those used by the paramedic. Except for suppression of warning dysrhythmias, most of the treatment skills are reserved for patients with symptomatic reduction in cardiac output. Particular care is exercised with defibrillation, due to the possibility of injury to others.

SKILL PROFICIENCY TESTING

Skill Application of Monitor Electrodes (Figure 6.56)

Performance Demonstrate how to apply monitor electrodes to obtain a modified chest lead on a patient with simulated chest pain.

Conditions
1. A patient volunteer will simulate chest pain.
2. A monitor will be available, for use by the rescuer.
3. A monitor cable with positive, negative, and ground electrode leads will be available.
4. Three electrode pads will be available to the rescuer.
5. Evaluator will tell the student to use the monitor cable to obtain a modified chest lead.

Standard
1. Rescuer follows the sequence in the Rhythm Monitoring Guide, making no more than 3 errors among the 11 steps. ☐
2. Time limit: 1 minute. ☐

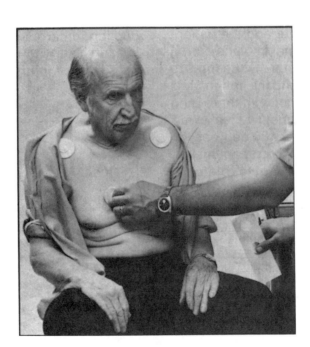

Student's Name _____ Date _____ Evaluator _____

Pass/Fail

SKILL PROFICIENCY TESTING

Skill Paper Readout (Figure 6.57)

Performance Demonstrate how to obtain a 5-second paper readout using a portable monitor defibrillator.

Conditions

1. The rescuer will have available a portable monitor defibrillator with strip recorder option.

2. The strip recorder will be empty of electrocardiograph paper.

3. The appropriate-size electrocardiograph paper will be available nearby.

4. An appropriate electrocardiogram signal will be available. (The evaluator may have a monitor cable attached correctly to himself or herself).

5. Evaluator asks for a 5-second rhythm strip to be obtained.

Standard

1. Rescuer follows the sequence in the Paper Readout Procedure Guide, making no more than two errors among the eight steps. ☐

2. Time limit: 2 minutes. ☐

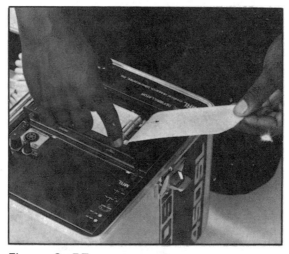

Figure 6-57

Student's Name _____ Date _____ Evaluator _____

Pass/Fail

SKILL PROFICIENCY TESTING

Skill Rhythm Recognition—Oscilloscope (Dynamic; Figure 6.58)

Performance Demonstrate how to recognize dysrhythmias generated by the Arrhythmia Anne and displayed on a nonfade oscilloscope.

Conditions
1. Evaluator controls the Arrhythmia Anne and varies the rhythms.
2. The rhythm must be recognized and orally interpreted in 15 seconds.

Standard
1. Sinus bradycardia ☐
2. Atrial fibrillation and/or flutter ☐
3. Atrial flutter ☐
4. Ventricular fibrillation ☐
5. Asystole ☐
6. Second-degree block ☐
7. Third-degree block ☐
8. Regular sinus rhythm ☐
9. RSR with PVC's ☐
10. Ventricular tachycardia ☐

Passing: 10 out of 10.

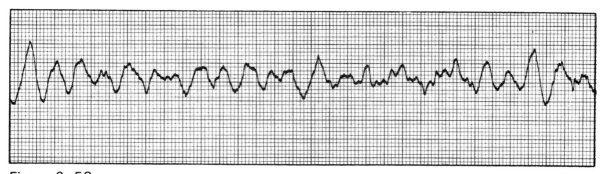

Figure 6-58

Student's Name _____ Date _____ Evaluator _____

Pass/Fail

SKILL PROFICIENCY TESTING

Skill   Rhythm Recognition—Paper Strips (Static) presented on EKG rhythm strips.

Performance   Demonstrate how to recognize dysrhythmias.

Conditions
1. Evaluator presents 15 rhythm strips to rescuer.
2. The rhythm must be recognized and orally interpreted in 15 seconds.

Standard
1. Normal sinus rhythm ☐
2. Sinus bradycardia ☐
3. Sinus tachycardia ☐
4. Sinus arrhythmia ☐
5. Wandering atrial pacemaker ☐
6. Premature atrial contraction ☐
7. Paroxysmal atrial tachycardia ☐
8. Atrial flutter ☐
9. Atrial fibrillation ☐
10. Premature junctional contraction ☐
11. Junctional escape rhythm ☐
12. Junctional tachycardia ☐
13. First-degree block ☐
14. Second-degree block—Mobitz I—Wencke-bach ☐
15. Second-degree block—Mobitz II ☐
16. Third-degree block ☐
17. Premature ventricular contraction ☐
18. Ventricular tachycardia ☐
19. Ventricular fibrillation ☐
20. Asystole ☐
21. Artifact ☐

Passing: all but 2 if 21 strips are used.
(Strips tend to be more variable than slides or commercially generated scope pictures. They are therefore harder.)

Student's Name _____ Date _____ Evaluator _____

Pass/Fail

SKILL PROFICIENCY TESTING

Skill Rhythm Recognition—Slides

Performance Demonstrate how to recognize dysrhythmias from a series of slides.

Conditions
1. Evaluator shows the student 13 slides.
2. The student has 10 seconds to see each slide and give an oral interpretation.

Standard
1. Agonal rhythm or dying heart ☐
2. Third-degree AV heart block ☐
3. Ventricular bigeminy ☐
4. Atrial flutter ☐
5. Ventricular tachycardia ☐
6. Atrial fibrillation ☐
7. Multifocal premature ventricular contractions ☐
8. Artifact ☐
9. Second-degree AV heart block (Wencke-bach) ☐
10. Second-degree AV heart block (Mobitz II) ☐
11. Ventricular trigeminy ☐
12. Ventricular fibrillation ☐
13. First-degree AV heart block ☐

Passing: 13 out of 13.

Student's Name _____ Date _____ Evaluator _____

Pass/Fail

SKILL PROFICIENCY TESTING

Skill Carotid Sinus Massage (Figure 6.59)

Performance Demonstrate how to perform carotid sinus massage on a patient with a supraventricular tachycardia which is symptomatic.

Conditions
1. A manikin with a palpable carotid pulse, IV line in place, O_2 in place.

2. An oscilloscope with monitor leads in place.

3. Evaluator should be able to input into the oscilloscope to demonstrate a supraventricular tachycardia.

4. Evaluator should say that the hospital has just asked the rescuer to perform carotid sinus massage for the supraventricular tachycardia patient.

Standard
1. Rescuer follows the sequence in the Carotid Sinus Massage Procedure Guide, making no more than 3 mistakes among the 10 steps. ☐

2. Time limit: 2 minutes. ☐

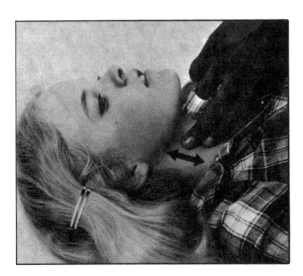

Student's Name _____ Date _____ Evaluator _____

Pass/Fail

SKILL PROFICIENCY TESTING

Skill Two-Minute CPR

Performance Demonstrate how to perform 2 minutes of basic CPR using both single- and two-rescuer techniques on a Recording Anne.

Conditions
1. A Recording Anne is available with plenty of recording tape.

2. The arms may need to be removed if they interfere with running of a long tape.

3. Although there is a team of two, only one person can get credit for the station at a time.

4. Rescuer starting first is told that he or she is the first to arrive at the scene where a patient has collapsed.

Standard
1. Rescuer follows the sequence in the Single-Rescuer and Two-Rescuer Guides (steps 6 to 12) provided, including one partner change during two-rescuer CPR. ☐

Student's Name _____ Date _____ Evaluator _____

SKILL PROFICIENCY TESTING

Skill   Defibrillation (Figure 6.60)

Performance   Demonstrate how to check a defibrillator, evaluate a patient for ventricular fibrillation, and correctly defibrillate when indicated.

Conditions
1. Portable defibrillator with paddle readout and paddle tester.
2. Gel pads for chest contact.
3. Arrhythmia Anne prepared for defibrillation.
4. Monitor cable plugged into defibrillator–monitor.
5. CPR crew available.

Standard
1. Rescuer follows the sequence in the Defibrillation Procedure Guide, making no more than 5 errors among the 21 steps. ☐
2. Time limit: 3 minutes. ☐

Pass: All critical steps, 12 of 16 steps.

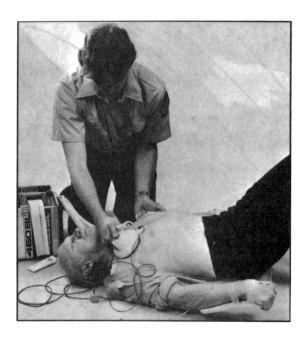

Student's Name _____ Date _____ Evaluator _____

Pass/Fail

7

Advanced Communications

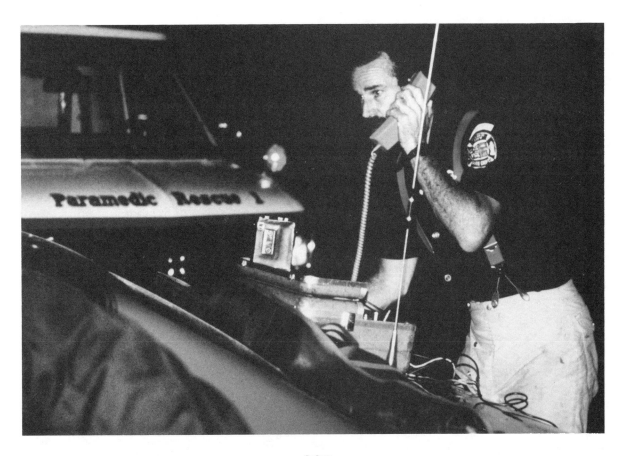

SKILLS OBJECTIVES

- **Radio Communication**—Demonstrate how to arrange material properly for radio transmission from paramedic to base hospital.

Outline

Advanced Communications
Skills Description

Skill Proficiency Testing

Advanced Communications Skills Description

INTRODUCTION

During most paramedic calls the paramedic must communicate with the following people: (1) the rescue coordinator, (2) the patient and/or family, (3) the other paramedic, (4) other fire or rescue personnel, (5) the base hospital by radio or phone, and (6) the receiving hospital in the emergency department. The communication described in this chapter relates primarily to that between the paramedic and the base hospital over the radio. The principles, once learned, will help with the other forms of communication.

Qualities

A good radio presentation must be short and informative, utilizing a format easily understood by nurses and physicians. It should include patient assessment as well as requests for therapy. Identification of the paramedic and the base hospital must be repeated with each order (Figure 7.1).

*This is a skills book. For parallel information as outlined in the Knowledge Objectives, read theory or assessment books.

KNOWLEDGE OBJECTIVES*

- **Radio Communication**—Identify the elements of a good radio communication to a base hospital.

Introduction
Record Keeping
Lab Practice

Comments

The conversation takes in its entirety just over 2 minutes of radio traffic time. The 3-minute pause does not tie up the air. This may be fairly long for such a straightforward diagnosis. The beginning paramedic student should be required to make such transmissions almost 100 times before starting to take shortcuts. As with the case of the patient exam, shortcuts taken early before the technique is learned leads to poor communication. Poor communication is the greatest source of error in the paramedic systems being developed. The argument that this radio transmission ties up other rescue conversations must be weighted against helping these students develop good habits.

Source

The format in Tables 7.1 and 7.2 is the method used by physicians to talk to each

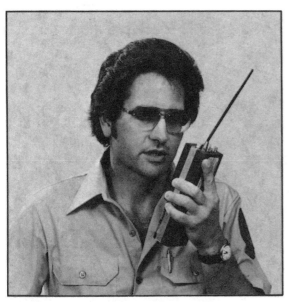

Figure 7-1 Communicate clearly.

other throughout the United States and probably the world. There is no good reason why physicians should learn to speak with paramedics differently than with each other except for eliminating rare, technical words and uncommon abbreviations.

Physicians also go through the stage of presenting patients to each other in great detail until they learn to be selective. Only after about 1000 presentations does the physician begin to get the right to take shortcuts. This pathway has stood the test of a field that is in all other ways changing. This is the pathway the paramedic and the mobile intensive care nurse should take in order to learn the skills of assessment and communication.

Table 7.1. PROPER SEQUENCE OF COMMUNICATION FOR MEDICAL PATIENT.

Goal	Speaker	Transmission
Paramedic introduction	P	Mount Diablo Base, this is Michaels 40 paramedic Brown with paramedic traffic.
Base hospital introduction	BH	Michaels 40, this is Mount Diablo Base. Go ahead with paramedic traffic.
Rescue, location circumstance	P	Mount Diablo, we are at the home of. . .
Age/weight/sex	P	a 62-year-old 70-kilogram male
Chief complaint	P	who was found by relatives lying unresponsive in his room.
History of present illness	P	He is a diabetic on insulin who missed lunch.
Past history	P	He has no other illnesses, other medicines, or allergies.
Medicines	P	
Allergies	P	
Overall appearance	P	On exam he has quiet, unlabored breathing, and is not pale. He arouses to mumbling when shaken.

Table 7.1. (Continued)

Goal	Speaker	Transmission
Vitals	P	Blood pressure is 130/80, pulse 120, strong and regular, respiration 24.
Head to foot	P	Pertinent findings include no evidence of head injury or Battle's sign. Pupils are middilated, equal, and reactive. Mouth is clear of obstruction. Breath sounds clear. Patient moves all four limbs symmetrically.
Assessment priority	P	We feel that this is a hypoglycemic reaction.
Plan	P	We are using left lateral position to maintain the airway. Would like to draw blood, start an IV D_5W, give 25 g of 50% dextrose, and if no response, 0.4 mg of naloxone IV push.
Medication order	BH	Michaels 40, this is Mount Diablo. We agree with your assessment. Draw blood as you start your IV D_5W and then give 25 g of 50% dextrose. Do not give naloxone at this time.
Medication repeat	P	Mount Diablo, this is Michaels 40. We copied order for drawing blood, starting IV D_5W, and giving 25 g of 50% dextrose IV.
Medication confirmation	BH	Michaels 40, this is Mount Diablo. That is correct. Proceed with the dextrose and let us know the effect.
(Three-minute pause)		
Report of medication effect	P	Mount Diablo, this is Michaels 40. We drew blood, started IV D_5W, and gave dextrose 25 g 50%. The patient is sitting up much improved, still somewhat dazed. Will transport to County Hospital Code 2. ETA 10 minutes.
Base hospital clearing	BH	Michaels 40, this is Mount Diablo. Well done. We will call ahead to County. KW1758.

Table 7.2. PROPER SEQUENCE OF COMMUNICATION FOR TRAUMA PATIENT.

Goal	Speaker	Transmission
Paramedic introduction	P	John Muir Base, this is Pomeroy 55 paramedic McGee with paramedic traffic.
Base hospital introduction	BH	Pomeroy 55, this is John Muir Base. Go ahead with paramedic traffic.
Rescue location and circumstance	P	John Muir, we are at the scene of an auto accident, 20 minutes ETA to Kaiser Hospital.
Age/weight/sex	P	Our patient is a 42-year-old 80-kilogram male who
Chief complaint	P	complains of chest pain and shortness of breath.
Background of complaint	P	The patient was the driver. He hit a telephone pole at approximately 30 miles per hour. He said he slammed into the steering wheel with his right chest. No external bleeding. No change in responsiveness.
Overall appearance	P	On exam he has quiet but labored respirations with early facial cyanosis. He is alert, oriented × 3. No wounds or deformity.
Head to foot	P	Pertinent findings include equal and reactive pupils, neck vein distension, tracheal deviation to the left, and absent air entry sounds on the right.[a]
Vitals	P	Blood pressure is 140/90, pulse 140, respiration 36.
Past history	P	He has no other illnesses, medicines, or
Medicines	P	allergies.
Allergies	P	
Assessment priority	P	We feel that he has a tension pneumothorax on the right.
Plan	P	We would like to use pleural decompression[b] on the right at the fourth interspace midaxillary line.
Medication order	BH	Pomeroy 55, this is John Muir. We agree with your assessment. Proceed with right pleural decompression, then follow with a trauma IV, keep open, started en route.

Table 7.2. (Continued)

Goal	Speaker	Transmission
Medication repeat	P	John Muir, this is Pomeroy 55. We copied the order for right pleural decompression and trauma IV, keep open, started en route.
Medication confirmation	BH	Pomeroy 55, this is John Muir Base. That is affirmative. Call en route to tell us the effect.
(Three-minute pause)		
Report of medication effect	P	John Muir Base, this is Pomeroy 55. The patient got immediate relief with decompression. Trauma IV has been started. Proceeding to hospital Code 3 with ETA now 15 minutes to Kaiser Hospital.
Base hospital clearing	BH	Pomeroy 55, this is John Muir Base. Well done. Kaiser Hospital will have a thoracic surgeon in the ER when you arrive. Call us back later for follow-up. KSP200

aPlacement of such important findings this low in the radio report is to show proper order of the complete report. With experience these findings should be given earlier in the report.
bNot allowed in California at this time.

RECORD KEEPING

Record keeping is done for many purposes:

1. Patient care
2. Teaching
3. Medical–legal
4. Billing
5. System evaluation

Every time a forms committee tries to come up with a single one-page form, these needs compete.

Types of records include:

1. Field notes
2. Paramedic field form (Figure 7.2)
3. Base hospital form (Figure 7.3)
4. Base hospital log
5. Base hospital tape record
6. Dispatch card
7. Dispatch center tape recording
8. Provider dispatch tape recording

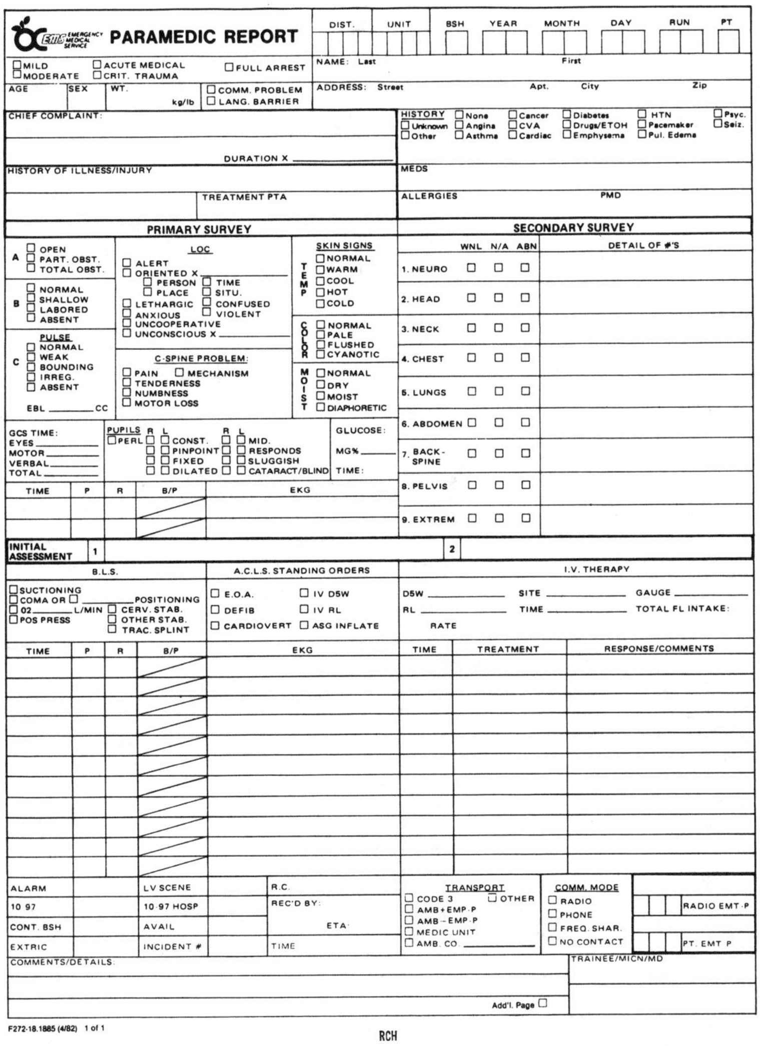

Figure 7-2

9. Provider billing form

10. EMS system form

The availability of this information to be shared among agencies is restricted according to the rights of patients to privacy.

The paramedic should learn the forms used in his or her system and practice using them during training. Good record keeping almost always parallels good patient care.

The base hospital run reports shown in Figure 7.3 provide a sample format for hospital records. Note the correspondance to the paramedic run report shown in Figure 7.2. The use of two pages is not as cumbersome for the hospital record as it would be for the field record.

Orange County Base Hospital Report

DIST.	UNIT	BSH	YEAR	MONTH	DAY	RUN	PT

NAME: Last   First

☐ MILD / MODERATE ☐ ACUTE MEDICAL / CRIT. TRAUMA ☐ FULL ARREST

AGE   SEX   WT. ___ kg   ☐ COMM. PROBLEM ☐ LANG. BARRIER

LOCATION (Incident): Street   Apt.   City   Zip

CHIEF COMPLAINT:

HISTORY ☐ None ☐ Cancer ☐ Diabetes ☐ HTN ☐ Psyc.
☐ Unknown ☐ Angina ☐ CVA ☐ Drugs/ETOH ☐ Pacemaker ☐ Seiz.
☐ Other ☐ Asthma ☐ Cardiac ☐ Emphysema ☐ Pul. Edema

DURATION X _____

HISTORY OF ILLNESS/INJURY

MEDS

TREATMENT PTA   CODE   ALLERGIES   PMD

PRIMARY SURVEY

A ☐ OPEN ☐ PART. OBST. ☐ TOTAL OBST.

LOC
☐ ALERT
☐ ORIENTED X _____
☐ PERSON ☐ TIME
☐ PLACE ☐ SITU.
☐ LETHARGIC ☐ CONFUSED
☐ ANXIOUS ☐ VIOLENT
☐ UNCOOPERATIVE
☐ UNCONSCIOUS X _____

B ☐ NORMAL ☐ SHALLOW ☐ LABORED ☐ ABSENT

PULSE
C ☐ NORMAL ☐ WEAK ☐ BOUNDING ☐ IRREG. ☐ ABSENT

C-SPINE PROBLEM:
☐ PAIN ☐ MECHANISM
☐ TENDERNESS
☐ NUMBNESS
☐ MOTOR LOSS

EBL _____ CC

SKIN SIGNS
☐ NORMAL ☐ WARM ☐ COOL ☐ HOT ☐ COLD
☐ NORMAL ☐ PALE ☐ FLUSHED ☐ CYANOTIC
☐ NORMAL ☐ DRY ☐ MOIST ☐ DIAPHORETIC

TEMP / COLOR / MOIST

GCS TIME:
EYES _____
MOTOR _____
VERBAL _____
TOTAL _____

PUPILS R L
☐ PERL ☐ ☐ CONST. ☐ ☐ MID.
☐ ☐ PINPOINT ☐ ☐ RESPONDS
☐ ☐ FIXED ☐ ☐ SLUGGISH
☐ ☐ DILATED ☐ ☐ CATARACT/BLIND

GLUCOSE:
MG%
TIME:

TIME P R B/P EKG CODE

SECONDARY SURVEY

	WNL	N/A	ABN	DETAIL OF #'s
1. NEURO	☐	☐	☐	
2. HEAD	☐	☐	☐	
3. NECK	☐	☐	☐	
4. CHEST	☐	☐	☐	
5. LUNGS	☐	☐	☐	
6. ABDOMEN	☐	☐	☐	
7. BACK-SPINE	☐	☐	☐	
8. PELVIS	☐	☐	☐	
9. EXTREM	☐	☐	☐	

INITIAL ASSESSMENT 1   CODE 2   CODE

B.L.S.   **A.L.S. STANDING ORDERS**   **I.V. THERAPY**

☐ SUCTIONING
☐ COMA OR ☐ _____ POSITIONING
☐ 02 _____ L/MIN ☐ CERV. STAB. ☐ OTHER STAB. ☐ TRAC. SPLINT
☐ POS PRESS

☐ E.O.A. ☐ ET ☐ IV D5W
☐ DEFIB ☐ IV RL
☐ CARDIOVERT ☐ ASG INFLATE

D5W _____ SITE _____ GAUGE _____
RL _____ TIME _____ TOTAL FL INTAKE:
RATE _____ ML/MIN

ALL IVS

Time Ordered	Time Completed	PATIENT EVALUATION					TREATMENT	CODE	COMMENTS	Ordered By
		P	R	B/P	EKG	CODE				☐ RN ☐ MD

F272-18-1884-2 (R4/84) 1 of 2

BSH COPY

Figure 7–3a

LAB PRACTICE

The skill testing sequence can be used by the student as a guide to the correct sequence for radio communication. Instructors may wish to give the students random information to organize into useful communications. Students working in pairs can critique each other. Once prepared, the student should dictate a presentation into a tape

Orange County Base Hospital Report

| NAME | | BSH | YEAR | MONTH | DAY | RUN | PT |

PATIENT EVALUATION

Time Ordered	Time Completed	P	R	BP	EKG	Code	TREATMENT	Code	COMMENTS	Ordered By
										☐ RN ☐ MD
										☐ RN ☐ MD
										☐ RN ☐ MD
										☐ RN ☐ MD
										☐ RN ☐ MD
										☐ RN ☐ MD
										☐ RN ☐ MD
										☐ RN ☐ MD
										☐ RN ☐ MD
										☐ RN ☐ MD

TRAUMA TRIAGE

☐ M.O.I.
☐ AUTO/PED
☐ EJECTION FROM VEH.
☐ SPACE INTRUSION
☐ THROWN FROM MOTORCYCLE
☐ FALL
☐ OTHER____
☐ FATALITIES IN ACCIDENT

☐ PENETRATING WOUNDS
☐ NECK
☐ CHEST
☐ ABDOMEN
☐ GROIN

☐ C/P DISTRESS
☐ C/P ARREST
☐ MULTI SYST
☐ CNS
☐ CV
☐ PUL
☐ GI
☐ GU
☐ SKEL

NEURO
☐ SINGLE SYST
☐ MULTI SYST

CHAMPION TRAUMA SCORE

		1ST	2ND

RESP RATE
10-24 = 4 PTS 1-10 = 1 PT
25-35 = 3 PTS 0 = 0 PTS
↑35 = 2 PTS

RESP EFFORT
NORMAL = 1 PTS
SHALLOW — RETRACT = 0 PTS

SYSTOLIC B/P
↑90 = 4 PTS 1-50 = 1 PT
70-90 = 3 PTS 0 = 0 PTS
50-69 = 2 PTS

CAPILLARY REFILL
NORMAL = 2 PTS
DELAYED = 1 PT
NONE = 0 PT

☐ GLASGOW COMA SCALE =

TOTAL
☐ CTS
1ST____
TIME____

☐ 2ND____
TIME____

ADDITIONAL COMMENTS:

☐ CONTAGIOUS DISEASE EXPOSURE REPORTED

SCENE DECISIONS
☐ INFORMED CONSENT
☐ IMPLIED CONSENT
☐ REFUSED CARE
☐ RELEASE SIGNED
☐ LEFT AT SCENE
☐ DEAD ON SCENE

TRIAGE DECISIONS
Code
☐ NEAREST R.C.____ ETA____
☐ BYPASS PER PT./FAMILY REQUEST
☐ BYPASS PER PMD REQUEST
☐ BYPASS OTHER (Detail)
☐ TO REGIONAL CENTER PER CRITERIA
☐ Burn ☐ Neurosurg. ☐ Spinal Cord
☐ Cardiac ☐ Pediatric ☐ Trauma
☐ Neonatal ☐ Poison ☐ Psyc.
RECEIVING HOSP.____ Code____ ETA____

COMMUNICATIONS
☐ RADIO ☐ COMM. PROB.
☐ PHONE ☐ NO CONTACT
☐ FREQ. SHARE

TRANSPORT
☐ AMB. + EMT-P ☐ CODE 3
☐ AMB. · EMT-P ☐ OTHER
☐ MEDIC UNIT
☐ AIR TRANSPORT   Code
AMB. CO.____

TYPE OF RUN
☐ BLS
☐ BLS & IV
☐ ALS

EMS OFFICE ONLY
(Leave Blank)
☐ SPEC. STUDY #1
☐ SPEC. STUDY #2
☐ SPEC. STUDY #3
☐ SPEC. STUDY #4

UNUSUAL SCENE ISSUES
☐ COMPLICATED EXTRICATION
☐ MD ON SCENE
☐ OTHER

TIMES		R.C. REPORT GIVEN TO:	ARN ON DUTY	SIGNATURE
OCC ALERT		☐ RN ☐ MD	BSH · M.D. ON DUTY	ARN
ARR. SCENE		INITIAL TIME: UPDATED TIME:		SIGNATURE
CONTACT BSH		EMT—P RADIO:	DETAILS:	M.D.
EXTRICATED		EMT-P PT:		
LV SCENE		TRAINEE/OBSERVER:		
ARR. HOSP				

F272-18-10B4-2 (R4/84) 2 of 2

BSH COPY

Figure 7-3b

recorder and later listen to it being played back. The student should be especially careful to paint the scene since the base hospital often misses the rescue circumstance in which the paramedic is working. The skill is further developed as the student starts working in the field under supervision where presentations are critiqued on a daily basis.

SKILL PROFICIENCY TESTING

Skill Radio Communication

Performance Demonstrate how to arrange material properly for radio transmission from paramedic to base hospital.

Conditions
1. The rescuer will be given a sheet of paper with random information.

2. After 2 minutes, the rescuer will be asked to dictate a radio presentation into a tape recorder.

3. Each student should have his or her own tape cassette.

4. A tape recorder will be available with a microphone with its own on–off switch.

Standard
1. Rescuer studies transmission for up to 2 minutes, and then dictates a transmission into the tape recorder. ☐

2. The tape will later be graded on the following elements:

Paramedic introduction ☐

Rescue circumstance ☐

Patient's age and sex ☐

Chief complaint ☐

History of present illness ☐

Past history ☐

Medicines ☐

Allergies ☐

Overall appearance ☐

Vitals ☐

Head to foot—pertinent ☐

Assessment ☐

Priority ☐

Plan ☐

Passing: 10 of 13 in correct order.

Student's Name _____ Date _____ Evaluator _____

Pass/Fail

Note: This format only standardizes the order of the communication. Subtle judgment issues can only be discovered from review of field tapes.

Index